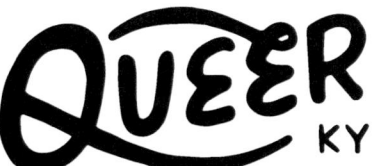

Queer Kentucky is a diverse LGBTQ+ run non-profit based in working to bolster and enhance Queer culture and health through storytelling, education, and action. Through our storytelling approach, we give visibility and celebrate the lives of LGBTQ+ people in the great Bluegrass State. Visibility alone is life-saving. Queer Kentucky actively works with organizations and businesses on their inclusivity efforts that enhance the well-being of their employees.

Dedication
To every Queer person struggling, and to all those
that have succumbed to their struggles.
Please know you aren't alone.

And to the thriving LGBTQ+ people and allies
working to enhance the lives of our community.

We see you fighting, and we're standing with you.

DONATE/SUBSCRIBE

Copyright © 2024 by Queer Kentucky
All rights reserved.
ISBN: 979-8-9880764-5-2
Queer Kentucky
PO Box 424
Covington, KY 41012

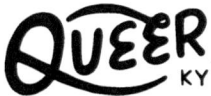

Executive Director
Missy Spears

Editor-in-Chief
Spencer Jenkins

Featured Artist
Jacob Grant

Contributing Photographer
Jon Cherry

Contributing Writers
Faulkner Morgan Archive
Silas House
Chad Kamen (UofL Archive)
Olivia Krauth
Cassidy Meurer (UofL Archive)
Belle Townsend

Design
Brackish Creative

Featuring
Cara Ellis
Carla F Wallace
Sarah Ratliff
Greg Bourke
Kaila Adia Story, PhD
Jonathan Coleman
Hannah Drake
David Williams
Tanner Mobley
Jaison Gardner
Chris Hartman
Shawn Masters
Anne Milller
Tyler Gabbard
Keturah Herron
Lisa Gunterman
Laura Petrie
Dawn Wilson
Julia Keister
Patti Minter

Web development
Honeywick

For advertising inquiries
contact@queerkentucky.com

CONTENTS

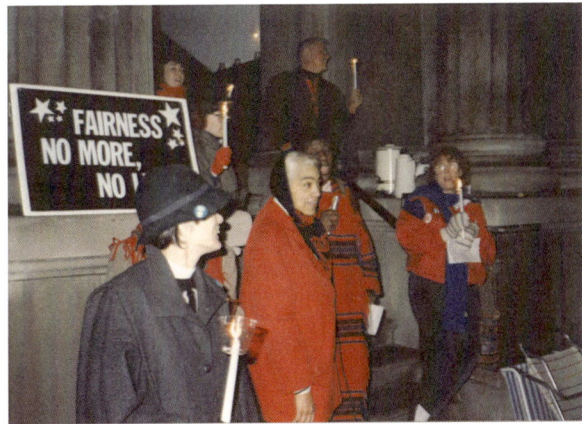

6
BUILDING PEOPLE POWER: STORIES FROM THE FIGHT FOR FAIRNESS

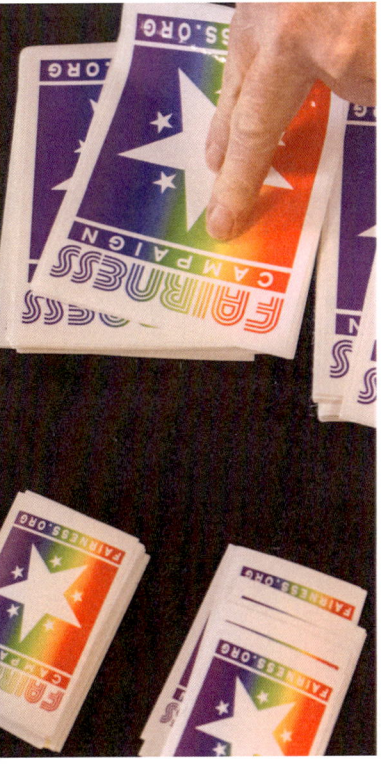

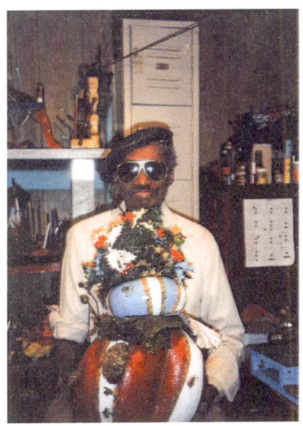

24
A COMMUNITY COMING TOGETHER: HIV/AIDS ACTIVISM IN KENTUCKY

40
WHY DOESN'T KENTUCKY HAVE A STATEWIDE FAIRNESS ORDINANCE?

54. TRAILBLAZER: KENTUCKY'S HIGHEST RANKING LGBTQ+ POLITICIAN, JIM GRAY

64. RELIABLY QUEER, SAFE, AND GOOD: DAY'S ESPRESSO AND COFFEE & MORE

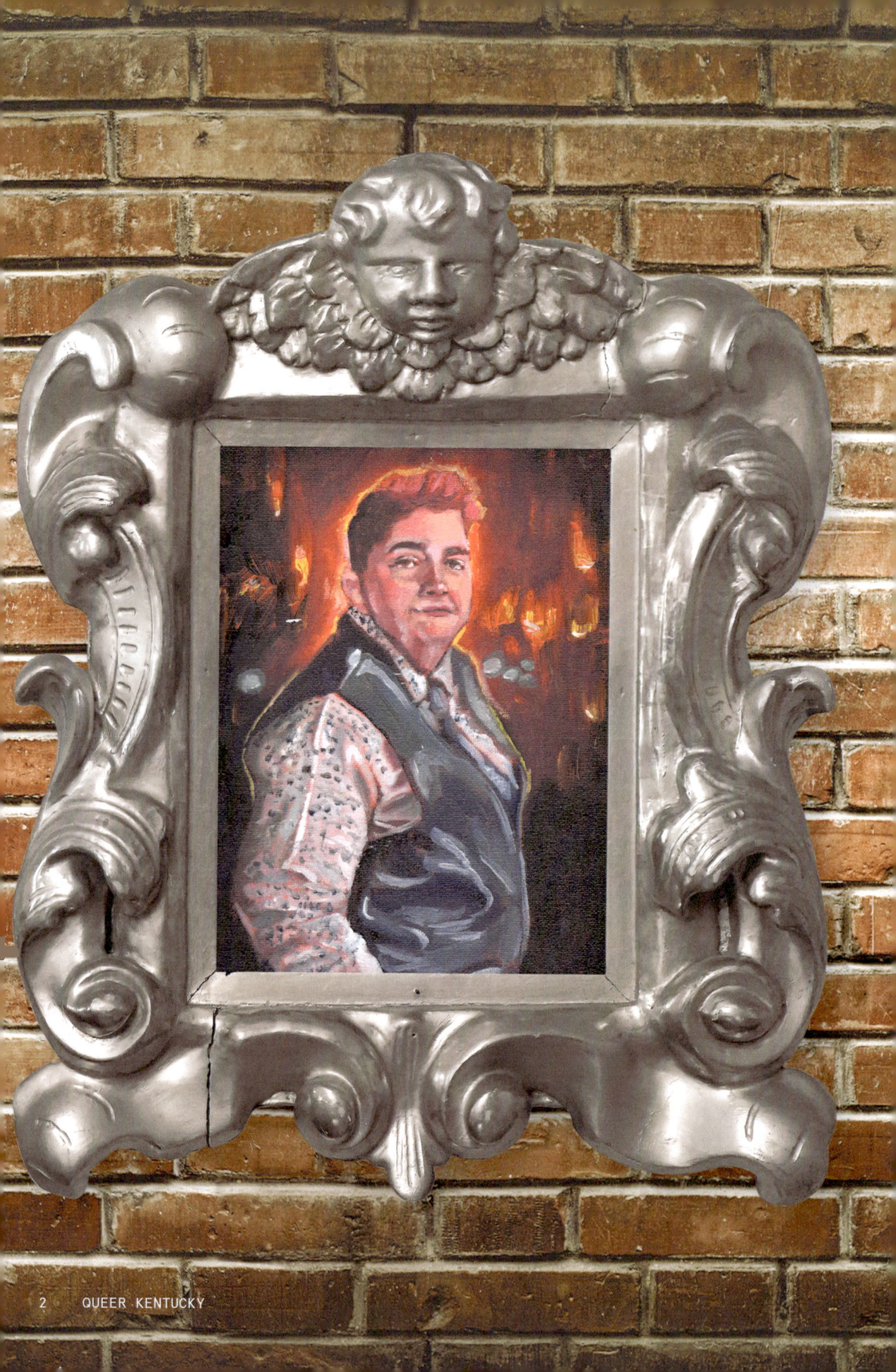

LETTER FROM THE EXECUTIVE DIRECTOR

Missy Spears

NORTHERN KENTUCKY

she/they   @missy.spears

"Caring for myself is not self-indulgence. It is self-preservation, and that is an act of political warfare." Audre Lorde

My journey to Kentucky was your common American dream.

Dyke lives in Ohio.

Dyke reads about a violent attack outside of a gay bar in Kentucky.

Dyke learns local ordinance makes this a hate crime.

Dyke moves to Kentucky.

The Commonwealth of Kentucky now boasts 24 fairness ordinances across the state and while no law can guarantee safety, justice, or carry the promise of enforcement, each of our 24 ordinances send a powerful message to our local community and statewide leaders. In its most basic form, each ordinance acts as a symbolic gesture (or warning) to local landlords, businesses, and residents. An unrealized and untested promise to take action "if" needed. At its best, an ordinance can lead to creating or scaling systems for enforcement so that when the need for action arises the foundation is already laid. And when over two dozen municipalities have to pass their own protections because the state can't, or won't, it sends a strong message to our elected officials that we can get shit done on our own.

Fairness serves as the legislative acknowledgment of the unique and often violent barriers that the LGBTQ+ communities face including higher rates of housing and employment discrimination, healthcare barriers, increased threats and acts of violence, and the overall toil that being constantly alert takes on your mental and physical health.

Our community doesn't ask themselves if they will be harmed one day.

Our community wants to know if they will be supported when it happens.

And that supportive web is growing. All across our Commonwealth are thousands of leaders working to expand Queer liberation in Kentucky by increasing community connection, education, access to resources, and advanced legislative protections. And it's a pleasure to be able to bring you a small sample of those incredible people, places, and history that have changed and saved LGBTQ+ lives across Kentucky.

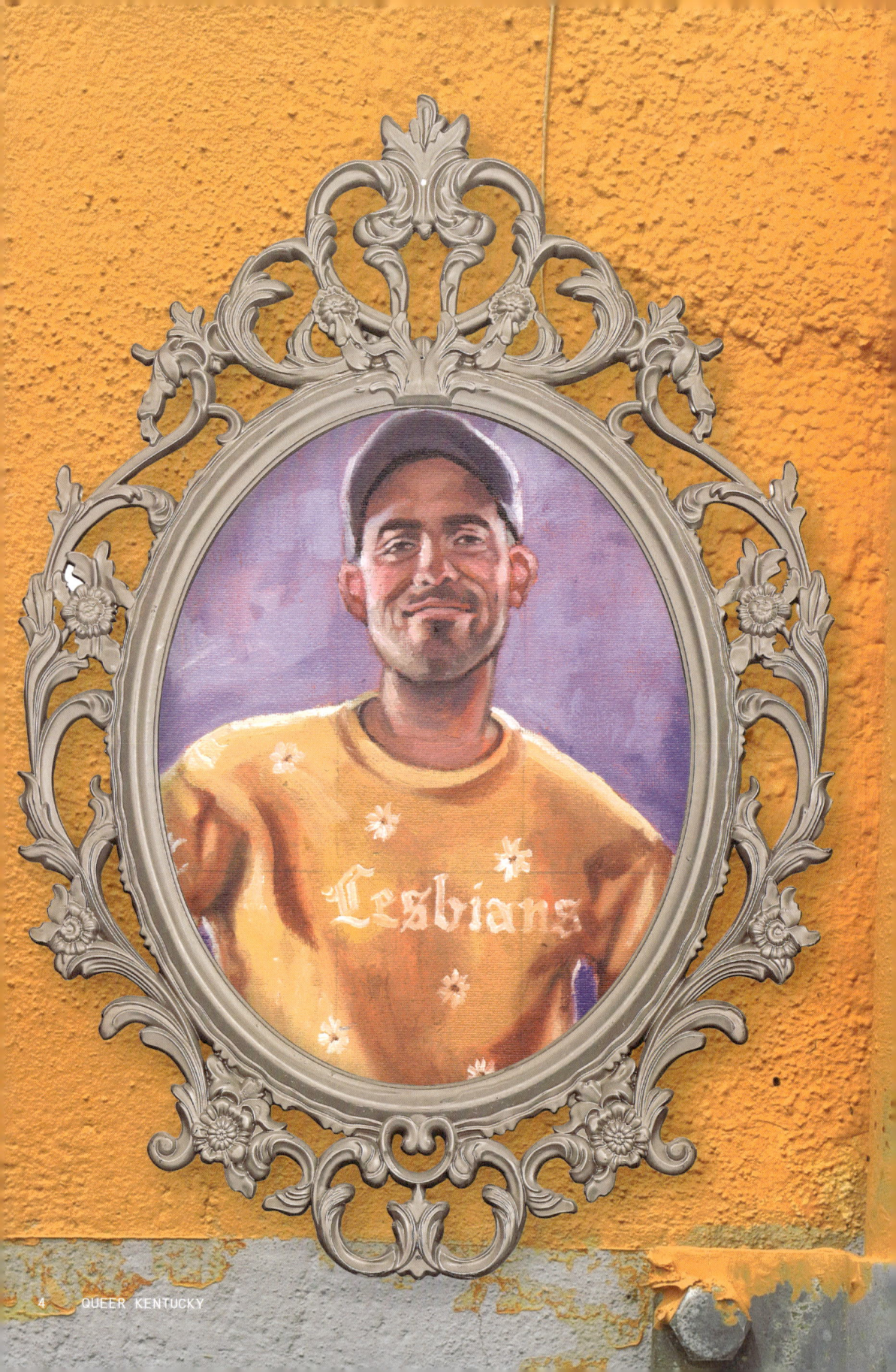

LETTER FROM THE EDITOR

Spencer Jenkins

LOUISVILLE

he/him   @spencerjenkss

Dear reader,

Countless faces, from Paducah to Pikeville, have played roles in advancing fairness and equality for the LGBTQ+ community across the Bluegrass — many of which proved foundational for my own path of Queer activism.

Ten years ago, I met Fairness Campaign Executive Director Chris Hartman for the first time at Galaxie, a swanky bar and restaurant in Louisville's NuLu neighborhood. I don't even remember exactly how we originally connected—probably just by virtue of being two gay men in Louisville, but I knew he was with the Fairness Campaign and I wanted to learn more about it. True to form, Chris rushed in wearing a suit and tie and slightly out of breath from running between meetings or perhaps from Frankfort.

I had just started writing for Louisville.com in an attempt to fulfill the city's need for Queer content. Ironically, I didn't know much about being gay myself. I had been out of the closet for quite some time, but struggled with and repressed my sexuality and Queer culture for years. Looking back, I think stepping into Queer journalism was my way of safely navigating an unfamiliar world through the lens of my work.

I rise to greet him, and of course I don't receive a handshake, but rather a firm Hartman bear hug that caught me off guard. Chris is a big dude with a big personality and I was still crawling in my skin as a shy gayby. I envied his confidence.

I was a sponge during our conversation. Chris filled me in on Bourke v. Beshear, the landmark case from Kentucky that would eventually pave the way for national marriage equality, which was already in motion. He opened my eyes to the discrimination and hatred faced by trans Kentuckians—things I had been completely ignorant to as a cis man. We discussed the anti-marriage equality campaigns spearheaded by Southeast Christian Church, and he handed me a roadmap of fearless Queer leaders throughout the city and urged me to connect with them. If I wanted to write about Queer culture in Louisville, he said, these were the people I needed to know.

I was introduced to names like Kaila Story and Jaison Gardner, whose Strange Fruit podcast opened my eyes to the Black Queer experience and what it meant to live at that intersection. I learned about David Williams, a renowned Queer Kentucky historian and archivist. And there were so many more—like Fairness co-founders Carla Wallace and Lisa Gunterman, to whom we, as Queer Kentuckians, owe an immense debt of gratitude.

Since that inspirational conversation with my now dear friend Chris a decade ago, hundreds of new activists have stepped up to join the fight for fairness and equality. Their dedication inspires a movement that continues to grow, but the work is far from over. We need every voice, every heart, and every hand to join us in this fight for a future where equality and justice are realities for all—together, we can make it happen.

BUILDING PEOPLE POWER: STORIES FROM THE FIGHT FOR FAIRNESS

Chad Kamen *he/they* Cassidy Meurer *she/her*
@uofl_archives
Special thanks to Pam McMichael for her help on this article

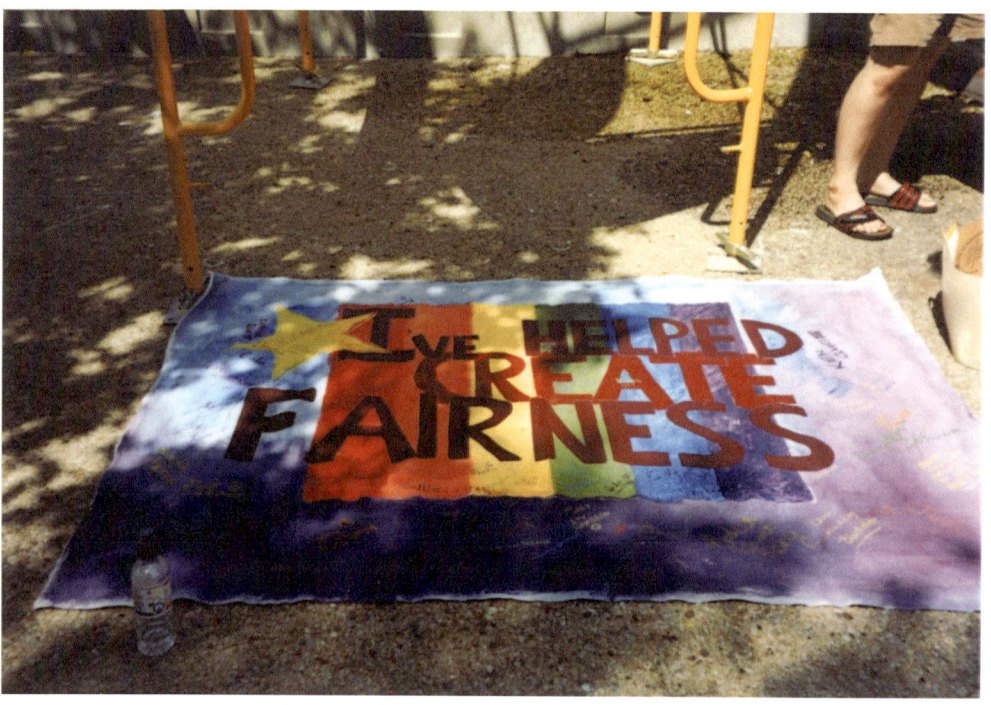

"I've helped create Fairness" tapestry on display, circa 1999-2000

Image credit: The Fairness Campaign records, Archives & Special Collections, University of Louisville.

SPARKING A MOVEMENT

In the mid-1980s, the shape of Queer activism in the state was rapidly changing. The onset of the AIDS epidemic, as well as changing ideas around visibility, mobilized organizers to focus on solidifying people power among Queer Kentuckians. An emergent activist group called the Greater Louisville Human Rights Coalition (GLHRC) followed this call to action in Louisville by pursuing anti-discrimination protections for Queer people. Their aim was the endorsement of the Louisville-Jefferson County Human Relations Commission, which they won in 1986 through documenting discrimination in the city and building coalitional support from civil rights leaders, such as Dr. Lyman T. Johnson.

Though the GLHRC was successful in getting an endorsement, there was a continued need for pressure to dismantle prejudice against Queer people, as well as to win the support for legislation from Louisville's Board of Aldermen. These continued fights led a group of organizers to create the March for Justice. As the first Pride march in Louisville, the march set the tone for activism in the area by highlighting the need for visibility, intersectional approaches to hate, and greater civil liberties. A key example of such was the march's connection to the passage of Louisville's Hate Crimes Ordinance. This intersectional piece of legislation, passed in 1991, was built in response to white supremacist violence against a Black family living in the Preston Park neighborhood. Through the coalition-building of activists across the city, the legislation became the first in Louisville to explicitly include sexual orientation as a protected class. However, the fight for clear and explicit protections against discrimination for Queer Kentuckians was just beginning.

CONSTRUCTING FAIRNESS

The March for Justice's 1991 platform included a demand that would become central to organizing across the state: the call for protections from discrimination in employment, housing, and public accommodations. To achieve this vision, organizers from the March for Justice and other related activist groups across Louisville established the Fairness Campaign, which would be formally announced during a press conference that fall.

From its founding onward, the Fairness Campaign served a variety of functions. It was an organizing collective, a community of friends, a support system, and an outlet for Queer expression. Built into the fabric of Fairness was also a call to anti-racist work, as the organizing team recognized that there could be no Queer liberation without that for people of color, specifically Black Americans. While this article focuses primarily on the Fairness Campaign's work toward anti-discrimination legislation, the organization's investment in anti-racism has been and continues to be substantial, ranging from trainings to internal assessments of organizational culture to coalition-building actions.

Building on the broad-based success of the Hate Crimes Ordinance, the Fairness Campaign was able to gain support for the first Fairness Ordinance in November of 1991. However, the measure never made it to a vote after support from the board began to unravel due to election turnover and homophobic external pressure. Following this attempt, organizers further committed themselves to getting the opinions of the board on record for future campaigning purposes. In the summer of 1992, the Fairness Campaign successfully mobilized support from the board for a vote, leading

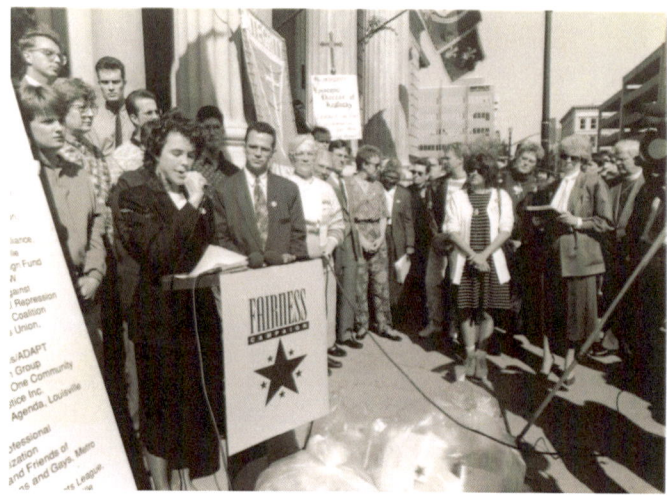

Carla Wallace speaks on the steps of City Hall during the Fairness Campaign's first press conference, October 9, 1991, Louisville, Kentucky.

to an 8-4 decision against the ordinance on August 25, 1992.

1992 also saw a transformation of the fight for Queer rights in Kentucky through the case of Commonwealth v. Wasson. Overturning the state's criminalization of consensual sodomy, the Kentucky Supreme Court's decision made the state the fifth in the country to strike down its sodomy laws. In turn, Queer organizers across Kentucky met this victory and the resulting attempts by state politicians to re-criminalize sodomy with fervor. The fall of 1992 would see organizers form the roots of what would the following year formally become Lexington Fairness and the more statewide-focused Kentucky Fairness Alliance (KFA).

With the goals of educating the public about LGBTQ+ issues and defeating anti-gay bills introduced in the Kentucky General Assembly, KFA pulled together a broad coalition of leaders from across the state, ranging from Henderson to Northern Kentucky. This building of unity would quickly be brought outward in 1993 through collaborations between KFA and the Fairness Campaign on an awareness-building booth at the Kentucky State Fair and extensive, successful lobbying in Frankfort. In 1994 alone, the political action committees associated with both KFA and the Fairness Campaign would defeat a slate of 15 anti-gay bills. By 1995, KFA built chapters in Paducah, Henderson, and Madison County, as well as developed a system called the Action Alert Phone Tree to mobilize supporters against anti-Queer legislation.

SECURING A FAIRER KENTUCKY

The mid-1990s saw new challenges in Louisville for the Fairness Campaign, as organizers encountered a generally unsupportive Board of Aldermen. In both 1995 and 1997, the Fairness Campaign was unsuccessful in getting an ordinance to pass, with both attempts involving restructuring of the ordinance's language in hopes of passage. While the effort in 1995 attempted to focus on employment non-discrimination, the 1997 push for fairness included the first fight to incorporate the language of gender identity. The latter push for the inclusion of gender was not taken up by Fairness's allies on the board for fears it would not pass, a move which would propel Fairness to deepen its commitment to trans solidarity in future efforts. In response to the unsuccessful attempts in 1995 and 1997, Fairness supporters engaged in civil disobedience by respectively refusing to leave City Hall and blocking Sixth Street.

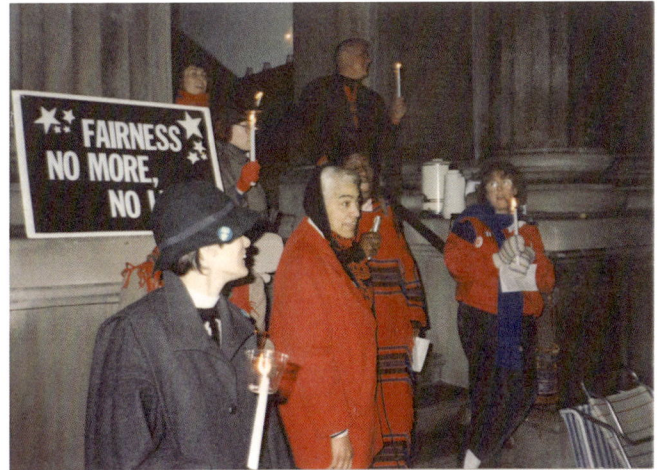

(From left to right) Sara Reed, Betty Payne, and Mattie Jones at a candle-light vigil for the Fairness Ordinance after it fails to get enough support from the Louisville Board of Aldermen, 1991, Louisville, Kentucky.

The year 1998 on both a local and state level served as a turning point for the fight for fairness. Starting this year, the Kentucky General Assembly would begin crafting and refining the Kentucky Hate Crimes Act. This act would become the first statewide hate crimes protection, as well as the first piece of statewide legislation to include sexual orientation as a protected class.

In Louisville, the discriminatory firing of Alicia Pedreira by Kentucky Baptist Home for Children would lead to a surge in momentum around getting an ordinance passed. Although Pedreira had disclosed her sexuality upon her hiring, her employer reacted negatively when an image of her wearing a shirt with the slogan "Isle of Lesbos" was displayed (without Pedreira's knowledge or consent) at the Kentucky State Fair. Pedreira's story broke through to the Board of Aldermen as a growing wave of news reports and Fairness-led events raised awareness about homophobic and transphobic discrimination in Louisville. The throughline of employment discrimination would prove successful, with the board passing workplace protections for both sexual orientation and gender identity on January 26, 1999, in a 7-5 vote.

The win in Louisville would usher in a wave of victories for additional communities in

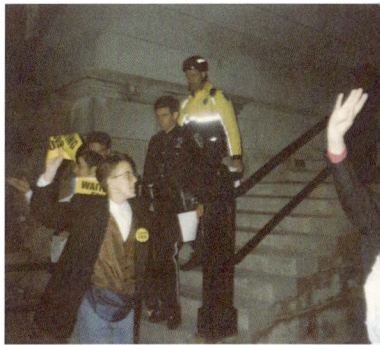

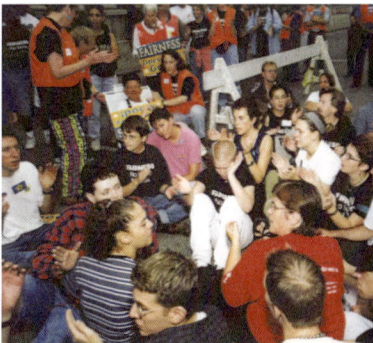

(Top) Fairness supporters and organizers including Lisa Gunterman (pictured on the left) leave City Hall under arrest, March 28, 1995, Louisville, Kentucky.

(Bottom) Fairness supporters block Sixth Street outside City Hall, September 9, 1997, Louisville, Kentucky.

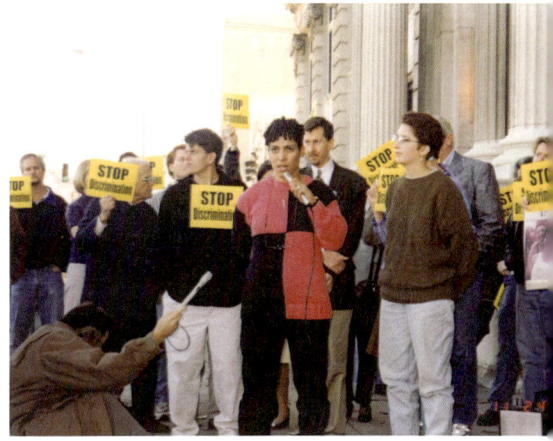

Alicia Pedreira and Faye Goodman address a rally outside of the Jefferson County Courthouse, November 24, 1998, Louisville, Kentucky.

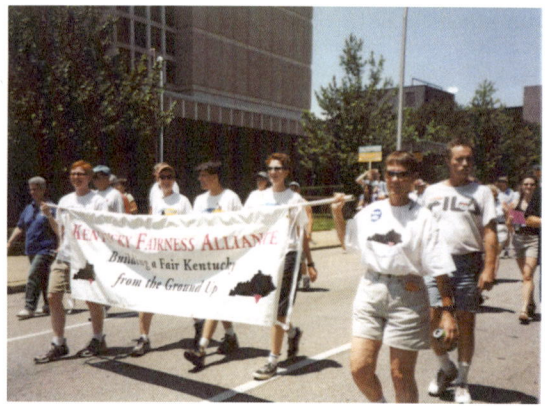

Kentucky Fairness Alliance at the 15th Annual March for Justice, June 24, 2000, Louisville, Kentucky.

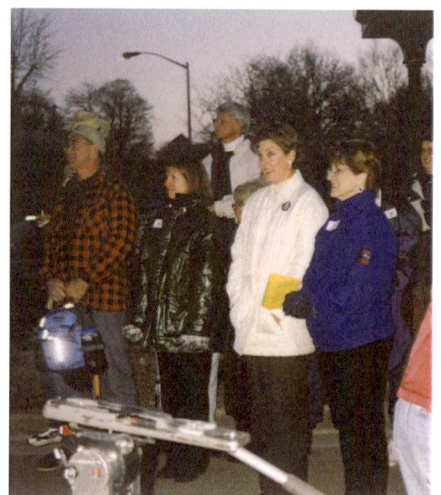

Kickoff event for the statewide Equality Begins at Home campaign, March 21, 1999, Henderson, Kentucky.

Kentucky. On July 8, 1999, organizers won the state's first comprehensive discrimination protections for sexual orientation and gender identity in a 12-3 vote from the Lexington-Fayette Urban County Council. The end of 1999 would also see similarly expansive victories reach Henderson in October and Jefferson County.

OVERCOMING OBSTACLES TOGETHER

For the Fairness Campaign and the Kentucky Fairness Alliance alike, the new millennium brought with it the hope of a more just Kentucky. Following the victories of 1998 and 1999, both organizations quickly found themselves navigating new terrain. The growing momentum for extending anti-discrimination protections to Queer people opened the possibility for a statewide fairness bill, with the first attempt at such being filed in the 2000 General Assembly. The four successes in getting ordinances also led to momentum for another win a few years later in Covington in 2003. The effort to get this ordinance on the books marked the first coordinated campaign between chapters of KFA to get comprehensive legislation passed on a local level.

However, the growth of the movement faced challenges. In Louisville, fairness Campaign organizers spent the first years of the 2000s focused on organizing against and then preparing for the merging of the city and Jefferson County. Merger, as it was known, created a different political terrain for activism, displacing power from the historically-Black neighborhoods of West Louisville to the often whiter neighborhoods of East Louisville. Changes in the government of Henderson also impacted organizers for Fairness in the city. After a successful effort throughout the 1990s to build community around anti-discrimination legislation, a new wave of city commissioners repealed Henderson's ordinance in 2001.

Coordinated backlash to greater protections for Queer Kentuckians would only grow in the coming years, as 2004 saw the escalation of efforts by state lawmakers to ban marriage equality. That year, lawmakers pushed for a full constitutional ban by putting the question of marriage equality on the ballot. The Kentucky Fairness Alliance and the Fairness Campaign joined together to defeat the measure. Through this effort, KFA and Fairness mobilized a network of over 2,500 volunteers across the state to get out people to vote "NO

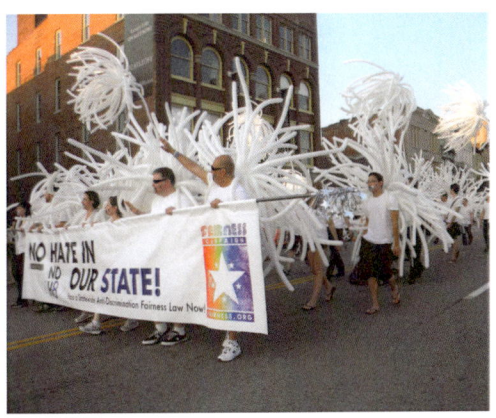

Fairness supporters marching for statewide anti-discrimination legislation in the Kentuckiana Pride Parade, 2010, Louisville, Kentucky.

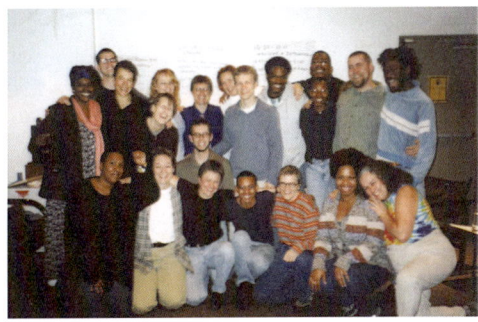

The Fairness Campaign team poses at a workshop hosted by Southerners on New Ground (SONG), circa late 1990's-early 2000's.

on the Amendment." Despite these efforts, Kentuckians would still vote the ban on marriage equality into the state's Constitution.

The bringing together of organizers through the NO on the amendment campaign led to deepened efforts at gaining protections on a statewide level, such as hospital visitation rights and partnership benefits for university employees. Collaborating on such a level also meant that organizers in the Fairness Campaign and the Kentucky Fairness Alliance needed greater structure for coordinating efforts, embodied in the creation of the Fairness Coalition.

A NEW ERA OF FAIRNESS

The 2010 session of the Kentucky General Assembly serves as a turning point in the history of the fight for fairness. It was the first in years to not feature any legislative attempts to discriminate against Queer Kentuckians. With the room to be on the offense, organizers could focus on shifting organizational strategies and structural capacities. After seven years without a new local anti-discrimination ordinance getting on the books, the Fairness Coalition decided to set their aims on the passing of new city ordinances.

To support these efforts across the state, KFA and the Fairness Campaign would slowly continue further aligning their work, ultimately merging into one organization - the Fairness Campaign as we know it today - in 2013. Their increased focus on statewide solidarity brought new faces and cities into the fold, including the Eastern Kentucky city of Vicco, which would become the smallest city in America to provide anti-discrimination protections for Queer people.

In its first decade as a statewide organization, the Fairness Campaign has focused on securing marriage equality, championing gender diversity across Kentucky, and fighting a renewed wave of anti-Queer (specifically transphobic) repression. As of July 2024, Fairness ordinances have now reached over 24 communities across Kentucky, ranging from Paducah to Morehead. Through the actions and organizing of Fairness Campaign team members and volunteers, the struggle for statewide non-discrimination continues on.

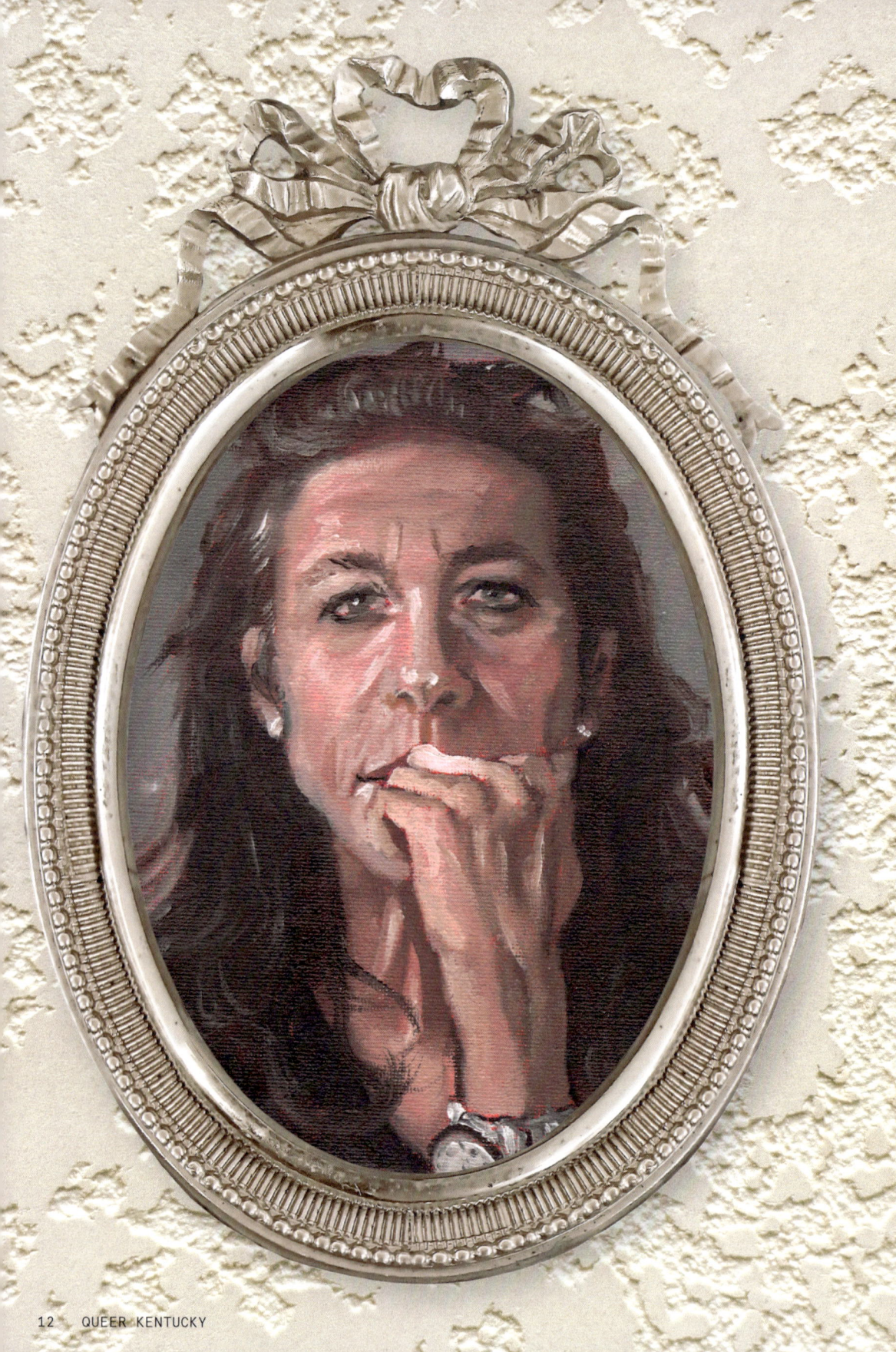

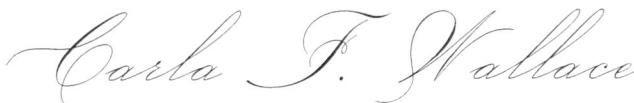

Carla F. Wallace

LOUISVILLE

she/her

Use one Queer slang word to describe Kentucky!

My partner and I say "Queebville" when referring to the Queering of Louisville.

How did you activate and organize your community for equality?

I co-founded the Fairness Campaign in 1991, which fought and won protections based on sexual orientation and gender identity in employment, housing and public accommodations in 1999. We centered racial and economic justice in that battle and made it a knockout, drag out public battle with protest, lobbying, public education, door to door work, civil disobedience and more. We refused to leave out gender identity, despite pressure from within our own LGBTQ+ community to do so, and won that before New York City and Chicago. We also used the people power we built to win place reforms and living wages for city workers.

In the last 25 years, what is one moment that gave you hope for Kentucky's fight in equality?

When so many Queer people who are white, joined us in the streets to protest when Breonna Taylor was killed by Louisville police. Only together can we win the world we need, for ALL of us.

What do you think is next for Kentucky in the fight for equality?

I want to see us on the frontlines in the fight for affordable housing, healthcare, and police accountability. Those issues have critical impacts on the most vulnerable in our LGBTQ+ community.

What are Kentucky's greatest strengths when it comes to the fight for Queer equality?

We understand that we have to fight collectively to build collective liberation. This is not about quietly trying to convince people in power to care about us. As Frederick Douglas said, "Power Concedes Nothing Without A Demand."

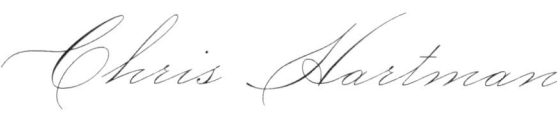

LOUISVILLE

he/him

Use one Queer slang word to describe Kentucky!

Girrrrrrrrrl

How did you activate and organize your community for equality?

I've tried to show up. In all parts of our commonwealth. I say, so much of the work is where we put our physical selves, or our attention.

In the last 25 years, what is one moment that gave you hope for Kentucky's fight in equality?

Vicco's passage of the Fairness Ordinance after a decade of drought was truly inspiring. While we knew it would become the smallest city in Kentucky with LGBTQ+ rights, we didn't know it would be the smallest in all of America to protect Queer folks from discrimination. That was truly magical, and the international media storm that surrounded it helped transform the conversation not just in Kentucky, but across America about rural LGBTQ+ support.

What do you think is next for Kentucky in the fight for Equality?

City number 25 with a Fairness Ordinance! (And maybe 26 & 27!)

What are Kentucky's greatest strengths when it comes to the fight for Queer equality?

Our grassroots organizing and support. The roots are deep in the Bluegrass.

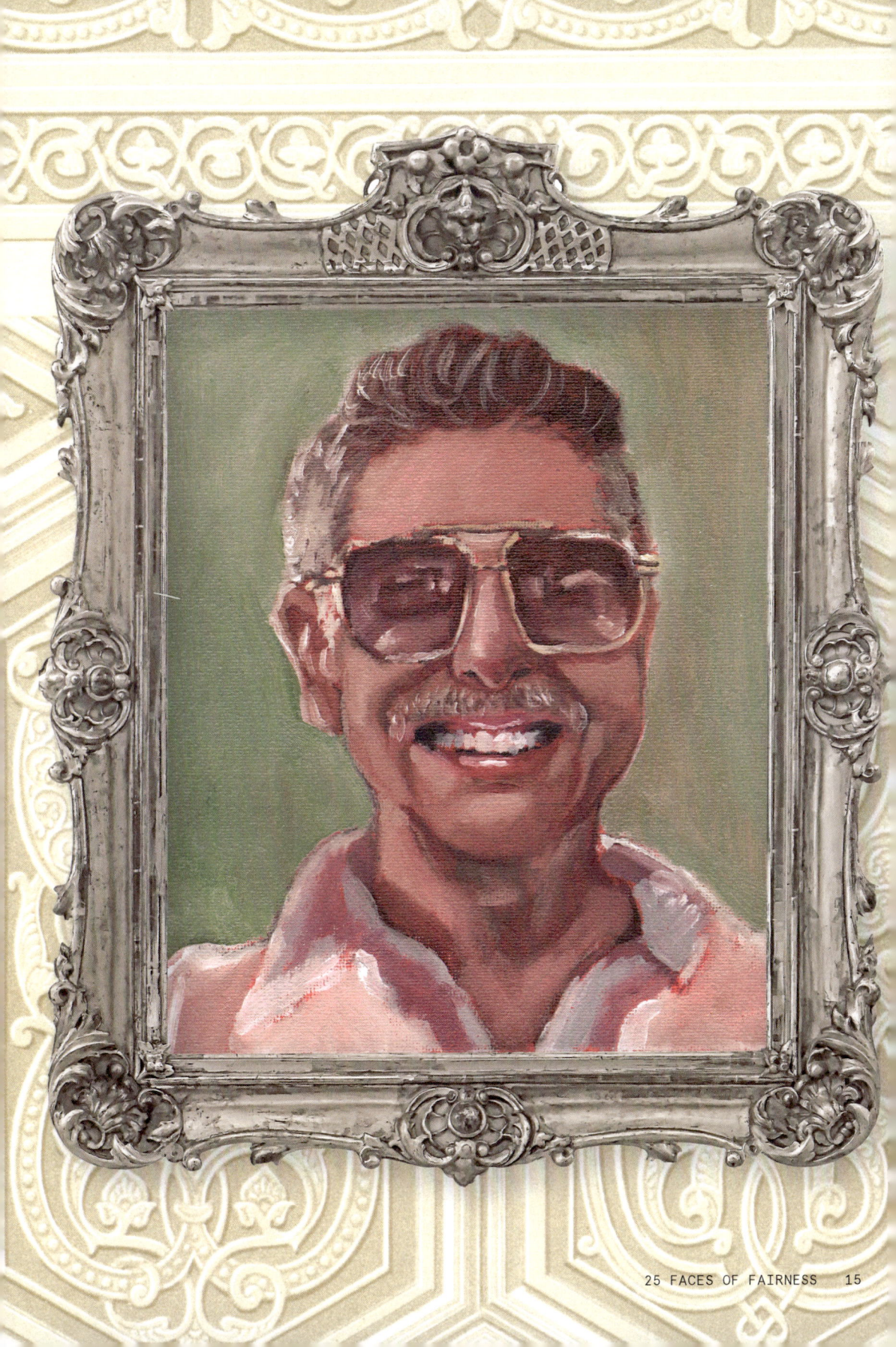

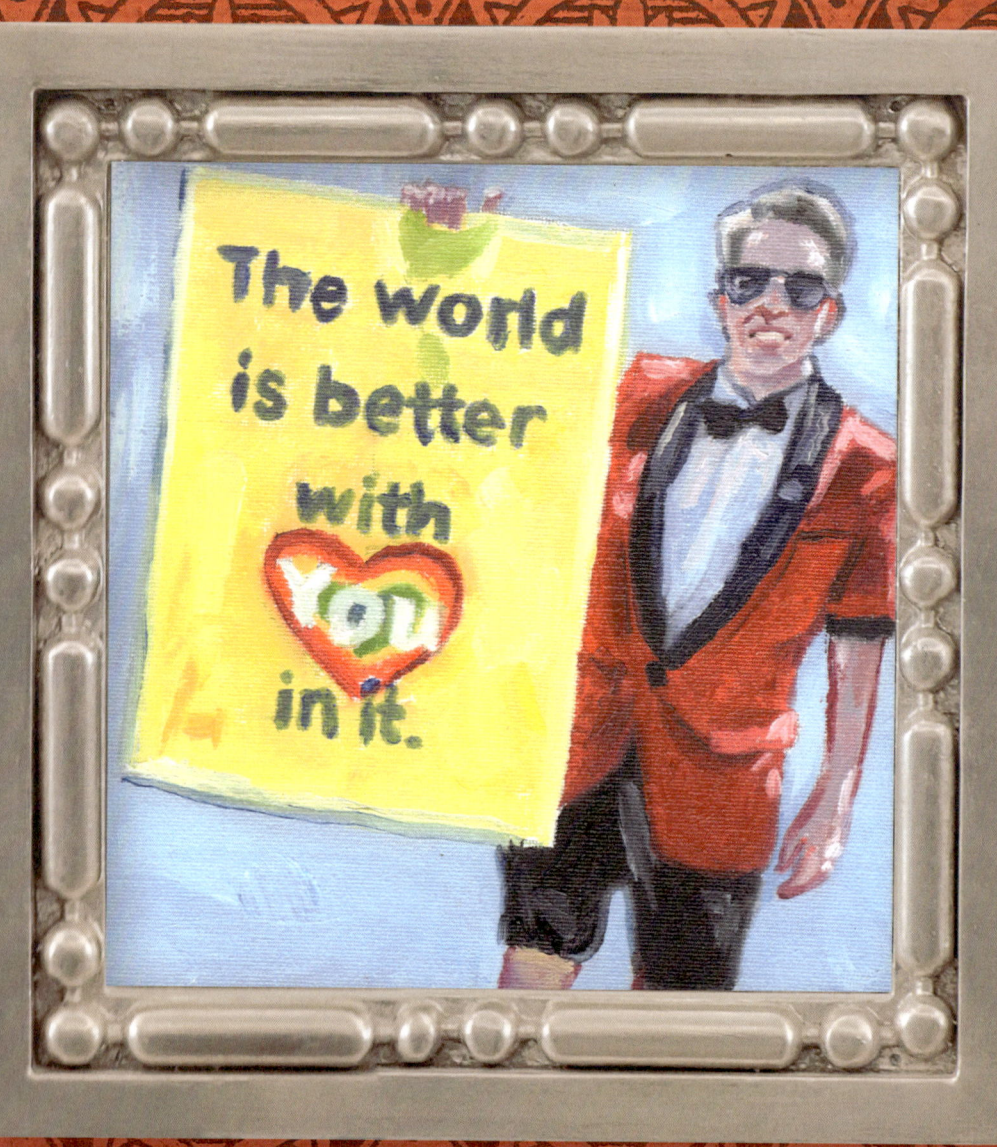

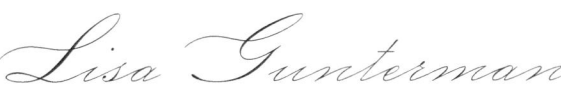

LISA GUNTERMAN
LOUISVILLE
they/them or "Lisa"

Use one Queer slang word to describe Kentucky!

Hot To Go

How did you activate and organize your community for equality?

We stand on the shoulders of giants. I have had the privilege of being mentored and supported by incredible leaders in Louisville's social justice and civil rights communities.

What do you think is next for Kentucky in the fight for equality?

We know from data that the current climate of bigotry is having a devastating impact on LGBTQ+ youth, including increasing their already high rates of suicide and suicidal ideation. This is unacceptable. We need more accomplices in the movement—including in the state legislature—dedicated to supporting LGBTQ+ youth and empowering them to not only survive, but thrive.

What are Kentucky's greatest strengths when it comes to the fight for Queer equality?

It is important to recognize that when the Fairness Campaign was founded in 1991, we founded as an anti-racist organization, and benefited from elders in the Civil Rights community, who served as our mentors and advisors. This intersectional approach is unique to LGBTQ+ organizations, and can serve as a model to communities across the nation.

Who is one other LGBTQ+ Kentucky leader that you admire and why?

I always say "the movement is collective," so rather than recognizing one person, I would like to honor and celebrate the volunteers. For more than 30 years, volunteers have driven the mission of the Fairness Campaign, advancing LGBTQ+ equality, first in Louisville, and now, statewide. Volunteers represented a diverse range of identities and took time out of their day to build a better world. Fairness would be nothing without the volunteers and I am forever grateful for their service and dedication to our community.

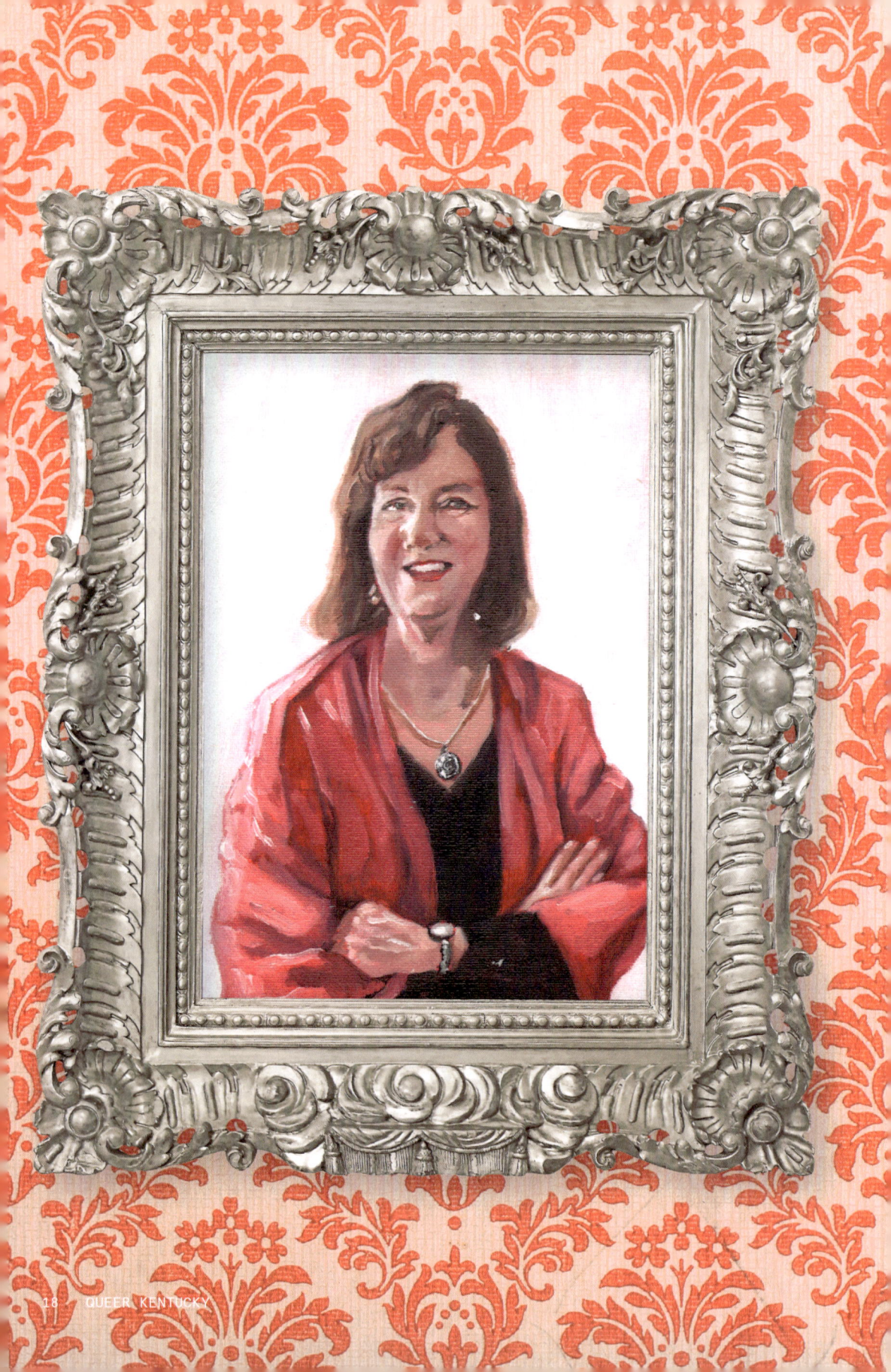

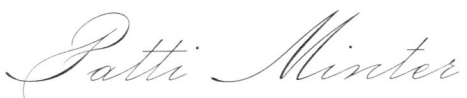

BOWLING GREEN

she/her

Use one Queer slang word to describe Kentucky!

Fierce!

How did you activate and organize your community for equality?

We started monthly Bowling Green Fairness meetings almost ten years ago to organize locally to pass a Fairness Ordinance in our city. From identifying LGBTQ+ supporting local businesses, strategy sessions, and meeting with elected officials to lobby them to pass the Fairness Ordinance, we built both community and power. We built a movement.

In the last 25 years, what is one moment that gave you hope for Kentucky's fight in equality?

In 2017, we tried to introduce the Fairness Ordinance at Bowling Green City Commission but failed to get a vote. At the next city commission meeting, Fairness supporters spoke truth to power during a work session and told commissioners why we desperately need this ordinance. For almost four hours, people came out on camera, shared stories of fear and discrimination, and spoke their truths in the public forum. Sitting there that evening, I realized that Harvey Milk was right when he said "hope will never be silent." I carry that with me every day.

What do you think is next for Kentucky in the fight for equality?

In 2025, Bowling Green, the third largest city in the state, will become the 25th city to pass a Fairness Ordinance. Finally.

What are Kentucky's greatest strengths when it comes to the fight for Queer equality?

Can't stop, won't stop. Year after year, I joined Queer activists and allies from all over the commonwealth and traveled to the state capitol for Fairness Lobby Day. Against all odds, people keep coming to their capitol to demand that their lawmakers see them and give them the rights that should belong to us all. In 2017, I led a group of Bowling Green Fairness activists to talk with elected representatives at the Capitol, where we were met with a chilly reception. Two years later, in 2019, the same activists came to my state representative office at the capitol and we celebrated what we can do when we realize that people have the power. I'll carry that tenacity with me to city hall, where I'll finish what we started 25 years ago and pass the Fairness Ordinance protecting LGBTQ+ citizens from discrimination in housing, public accommodations, and employment.

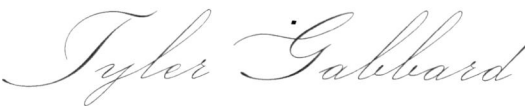

BELLEVUE/COVINGTON

he/him

Use one Queer slang word to describe Kentucky!

Confirmed Bachelor

How did you activate and organize your community for equality?

Representation—both in the stories we tell and the artists we work with on stage and off—is central to my work as a producer. I'm committed to bringing at least one meaningful Queer story to our audiences each season and to hiring artists who can tell the story with authenticity. Our audiences are growing and becoming more diverse as a result. Seeing the profound impact these shows have on our audience is worth whatever pushback we've gotten. It's also given us the opportunity to partner with some amazing organizations in our community who are on the frontline of the fight for equality.

In the last 25 years, what is one moment that gave you hope for Kentucky's fight in equality?

Year after year, I'm given a new jolt of hope at the NKY Pride Parade and Festival. It continues to grow but remains firmly rooted in the community with a wide range of local organizations represented. Having grown up here, it's always exciting to see familiar faces at Pride for the first time. The individual, personal change that happens at this level builds the foundation for big, sweeping change.

What are Kentucky's greatest strengths when it comes to the fight for Queer equality?

Kentucky's artists and creatives (especially drag performers!) are leading voices in the fight for equality. They're quick to give their time and talents to the cause. Our arts organizations engage with themes of diversity and inclusion and champion Queer stories. This work is pivotal in fostering broader acceptance and in building resources for the activists and nonprofits leading the fight.

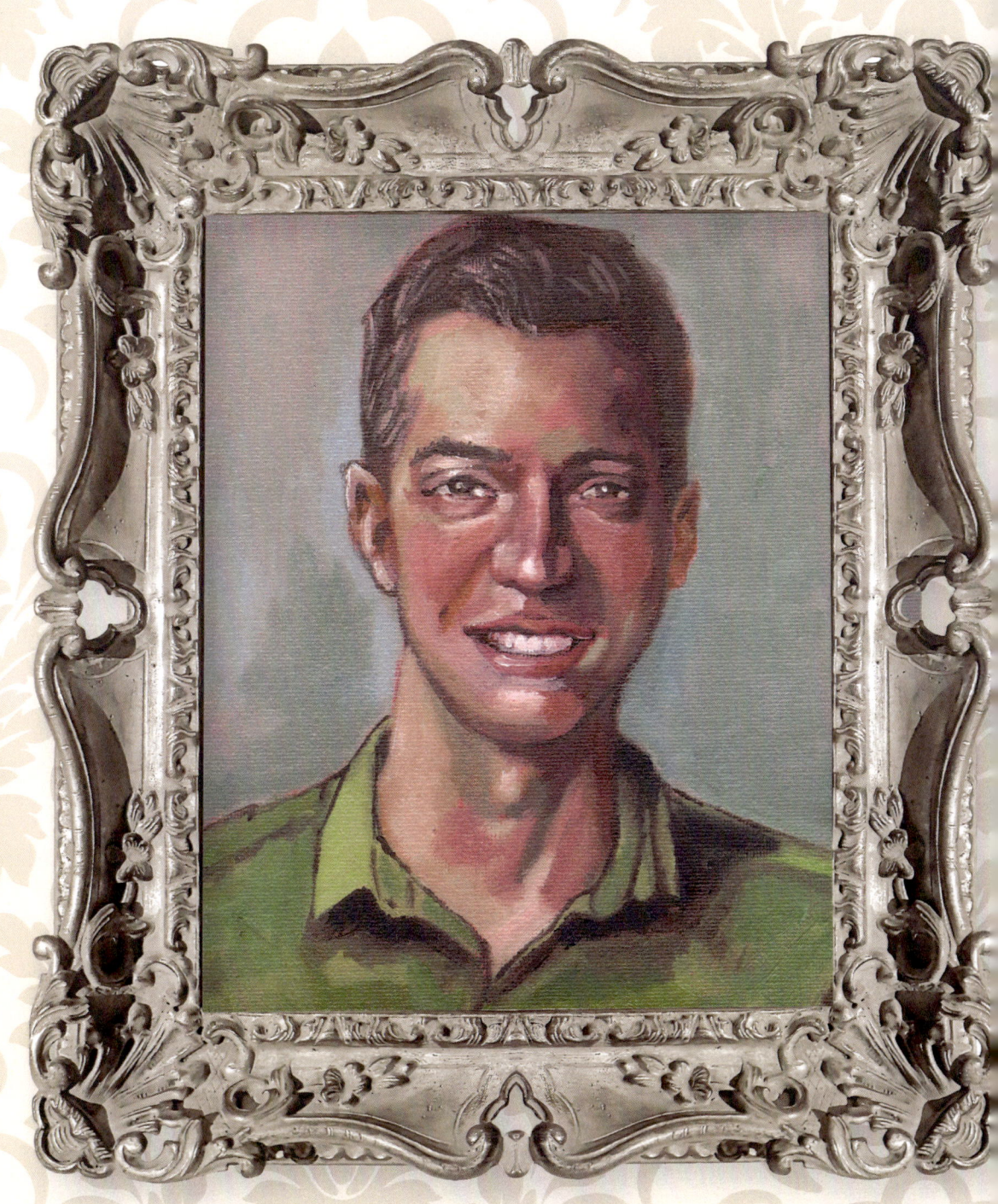

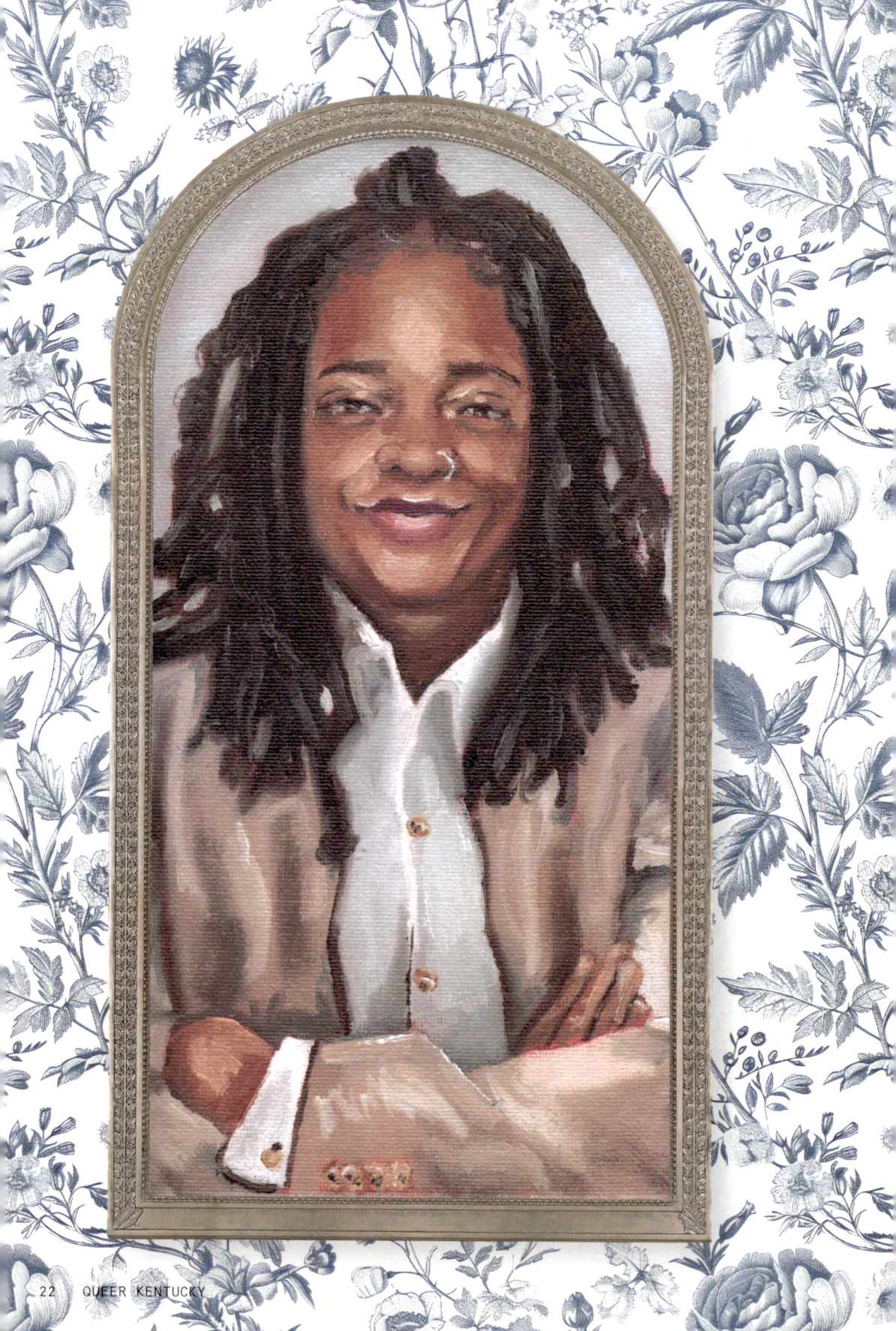

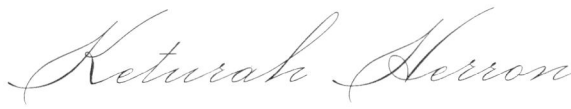

Keturah Herron

LOUISVILLE

she/they

Use one Queer slang word to describe Kentucky!

Stud

How did you activate and organize your community for equality?

Historically, most of the organizing I have done is around voter registration and GOTV. However, in 2020 I worked to pass Breonna's Law—banning no-knock warrants—through the Louisville Metro Council in just 17 days. Less than a year later, I played a pivotal role in putting together a bipartisan coalition to pass a statewide ban on no-knock warrants in the General Assembly.

In the last 25 years, what is one moment that gave you hope for Kentucky's fight in equality?

In 2023, so many youth organized and mobilized themselves to have a presence in Frankfort. They came to the Capitol and used their voices to speak against inequality and hate directed towards trans youth. I remember being encouraged and inspired by their bravery and courage. They were bold, loud, and proud. They showed signs of not backing down. We as adults can learn from them.

What do you think is next for Kentucky in the fight for equality?

The fight in Kentucky is the same as it always has been. However, I believe leaders like myself have to prioritize making room for youth. We must teach them, train them, and allow them to walk beside us as we fight. The Commonwealth which we are fighting for doesn't belong to us anymore. It belongs to the youth.

What are Kentucky's greatest strengths when it comes to the fight for Queer equality?

The biggest strength we have is history. There are people who have been fighting long before me. We must learn from our history. We must understand the fight is the same. We must be willing to relinquish our power to the next generation and make room for them.

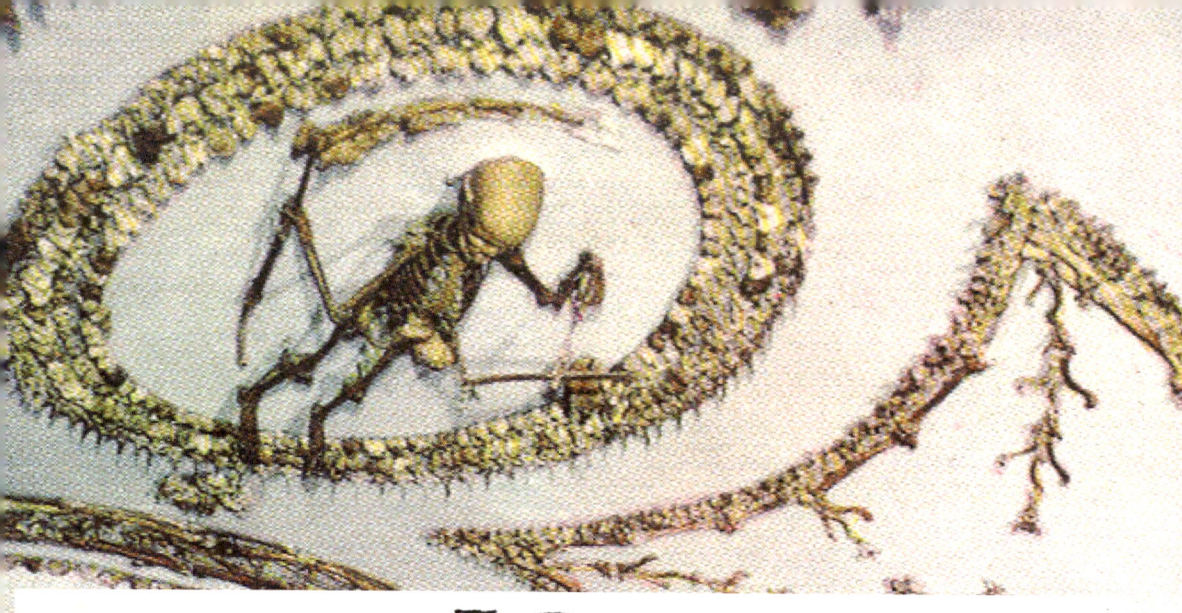

ROMA - Via Veneto, 27
Cimitero dei Cappuccini - 5ª Cappella
Cemetery of Capuchins - 5th Chapel
Cimetière des Capucins - 5ème Chapelle
Friedhof der Kapuziner - Fünfte Kapelle

Shall we start worring about AIDS? Chris fell down drunk in his gown on the 4th of July. Bradley is sueing his family. The more things change the more they stay the same.

Bob Morgan
628 NC
Lakeworth, Fla.
33460

Front (behind) and Back of Postcard from Frank Close to Bob Morgan, depicting the crypt of Capuchin monks in Rome, July 14, 1983, Collection of Faulkner Morgan Archive.

A COMMUNITY COMING TOGETHER: HIV/AIDS ACTIVISM IN KENTUCKY

FAULKNER MORGAN ARCHIVE
@faulknermorganarchive

In 1983, Lexington artist Frank Close sent a postcard from Lexington to the artist Robert Morgan, who was living in Florida at the time. The first line, casually, reads "shall we start to worry about AIDS?" The postcard, almost prophetic, depicts the crypt of Capuchin monks in Rome. As if Close's postcard was a sign of what was to come, the bodies did indeed pile up. Queer people across Kentucky would be lost and, while the exact numbers are still not known, it is certainly in the thousands.

Going back a few years to the 1970s, after the Stonewall riots, the sky really seemed the limit for LGBTQ+ people. The tides had begun to shift, and the Queer community was demanding space in society. But as the 1980s progressed, a dark cloud was on the horizon. At first it seemed so distant, just a blip on the screen—a rare disease, "a gay cancer," popping up in major American cities.

When we talk about the devastating impact of the HIV/AIDS epidemic, the story is often told through urban centers like New York City and San Francisco. However, this impact reached throughout the country and was just as prevalent and crippling here in the Bluegrass state—perhaps even more so. At the Faulkner Morgan Archive, we have been particularly keen to record the stories of this lost generation.

At this time, though, there was this deep connection between Kentucky and those major metropolitan centers. Many Queer individuals moved out of Kentucky in pursuit of their dreams, and ended up in the "gayborhoods" of cities like NYC. Shea Metcalf, who moved to New York City in the 1970s, grew up in Lancaster. Through his modeling career, he soon became friends with legendary artists such as Paul Cadmus, Keith Haring, Jean-Michel Basquiat, and Andy Warhol. Being in NYC during the height of the epidemic, though, Shea sadly passed away in 1991 due to AIDS complications, preceded by his boyfriend Drew Holbrook in 1990, and was later buried in his hometown.

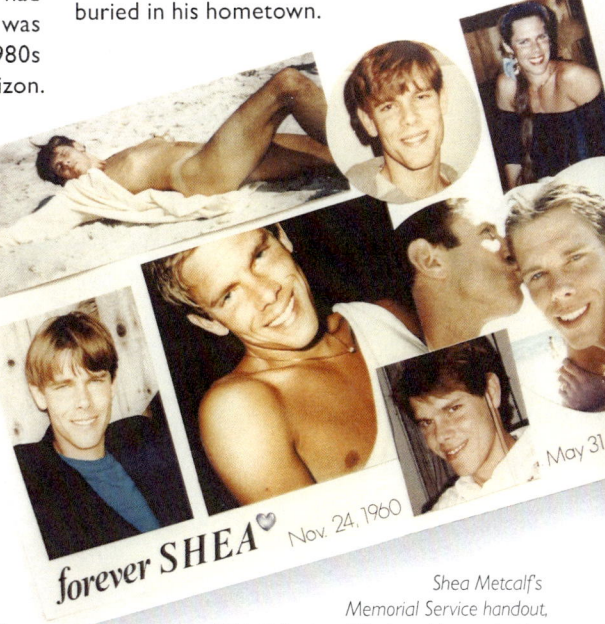

Shea Metcalf's Memorial Service handout, 1991, Collection of Faulkner Morgan Archive.

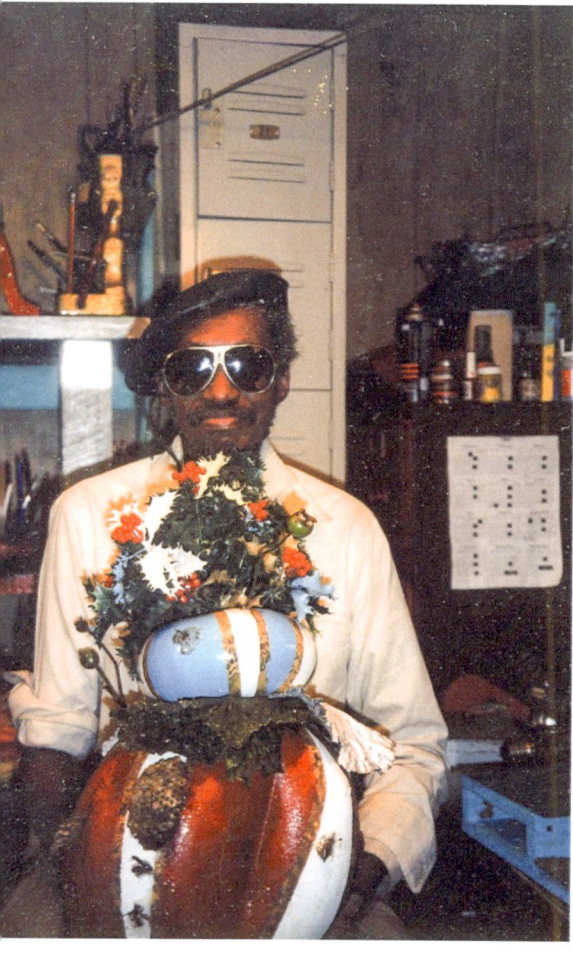

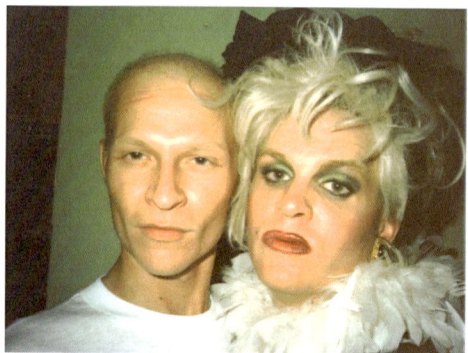

Darryl Brannock (top) and Chris Sloane (aka Christina Serpentina) (right), photo by Bob Morgan, circa 1987, Collection of Faulkner Morgan Archive.

Charles Williams in his home in Lexington, Photo by Robert Morgan, Date unknown, Collection of Faulkner Morgan Archive.

Local Queer folks, even those who participated very little in earlier gay liberation movements, become extraordinarily politicized in the midst of the devastation of AIDS. Friends became caretakers, and strangers became patients. Darryl Brannock was the first Lexingtonian to go public with HIV/AIDS and, in 1986, was likely the first Kentuckian to begin receiving AZT medications.

The HIV/AIDS epidemic was especially hard on communities of color due to the overlapping of homophobia and racism. One local artist, Charles Williams, dealt with this firsthand. Born in Blue Diamond, Kentucky, Williams worked avidly on paintings, drawings, assemblages, sculptures, and furniture until his untimely death in 1998, the result of AIDS-related complications and starvation. Along with the difficulty of living with HIV/AIDS, there was also simply a lack of widespread support for those suffering. Those in our community who became caretakers were stretched thin trying to battle the overwhelming devastation of the crisis.

The LGBTQ+ community of Kentucky mourned their dead, both near and far, and fought the disease as best they could. Despite these important and sometimes life-saving efforts, Lexington was also a difficult place to be during AIDS. The local police began enforcing the sodomy laws in a much more draconian fashion—a direct response to the local fear of AIDS.

In 1986, during an entrapment sting in the back parking lot of The Bar Complex in Lexington

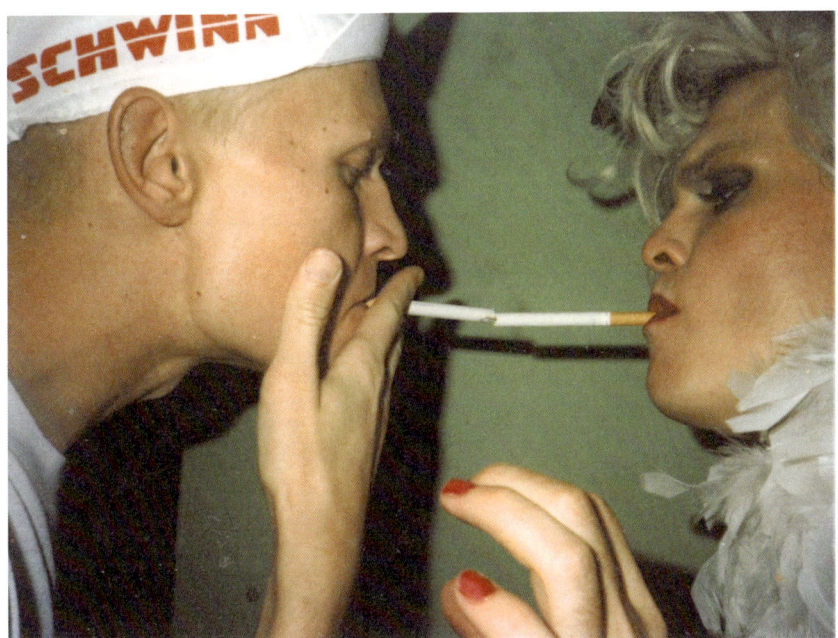

(the oldest continuous LGBTQ+ gathering place in Kentucky), numerous men were arrested, including a young nurse from Stanton—Jeffery Wasson. Wasson refused to quietly go along, challenging his arrest. Although his case lasted seven years, defended by a group of local lawyers, Wasson's defiance led to the overturn of Kentucky's sodomy laws, making us the first state to do so after the advent of AIDS.

As an inadvertent result of the HIV/AIDS epidemic, there was a major mobilization that happened in the LGBTQ+ community. Before the late 1980s and early 1990s, the idea of being part of an "LGBTQ+" community was not an understood part of being a Queer person. However, in the face of such a devastating disease that showed the disdain of the U.S. government, Queer people realized that no one else would care for them except each other. There was a huge shift with the Queer community coming together which was not there before. Having to literally fight for your lives does that to a group of people.

Grassroots activism began to turn into official organizations and nonprofits, many of which are still helping Kentucky communities today. Political conversations grew, especially the desire for basic protections under the law, such as not being fired or thrown out of housing because of one's sexual orientation or gender expression.

After years of activism throughout the 1990s, Louisville became the first city in Kentucky to protect its gay and lesbian citizens through the Fairness Ordinance, passed on January 26, 1999. Although the ordinance did not protect gender expression for trans Kentuckians until later, it was a major step in LGBTQ+ rights. A few months later, on July 8, Lexington became the second city in Kentucky to pass a Fairness Ordinance, and the first to include trans people in the ordinance. Now, a growing number of cities across the Commonwealth have passed Fairness ordinances protecting Queer Kentuckians.

These stories not only represent the national and international connections of Kentucky's Queer community, but are also a testament to all those who were lost in the AIDS crisis. The modern successes in HIV/AIDS prevention serve as a celebration of their legacy. We are now the bearers of their stories and the continuation of their activism.

nymph(o)

queer, sex-positive magazine

nymphomagzine.info@gmail.com
nymphomagzine.com
@nympho.magazine

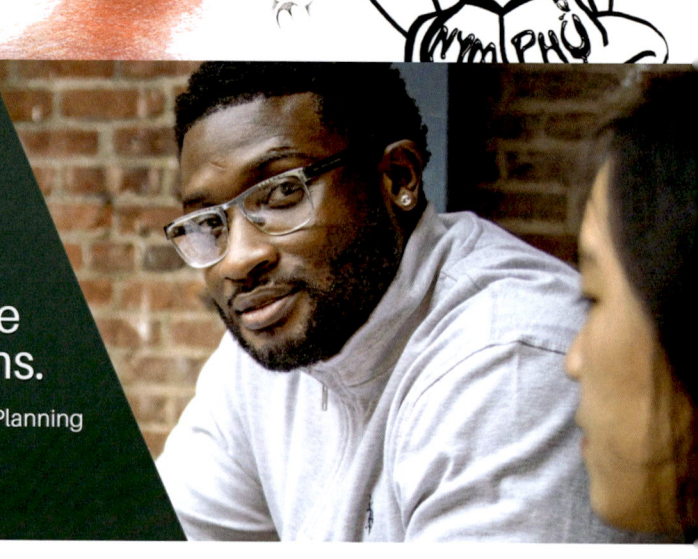

GRIMES
AND ASSOCIATES, LLC

We love working with dreamers, even if you use a different word for dreams.

Bookkeeping | Financial Consulting | Payroll | Tax Planning

grimesandassociatesllc.com

Business support that meets you where you are! ✨

Inclusive and training-focused business support

Website Design | Branding Design
Graphic Design | Marketing Support

Alight Agency is Queer, Appalachian, and Woman Owned, ready to help you run your business with confidence and joy. ✨

AlightAgency.com | @AlightAgency | (859) 351-3542

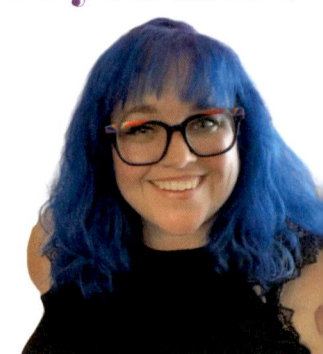

YOUR LOCAL HUB FOR LGBTQIA SUPPORT AND COMMUNITY RESOURCES

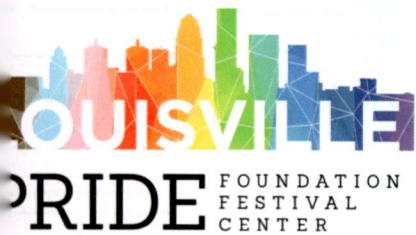

LOUISVILLE PRIDE FOUNDATION FESTIVAL CENTER

LOUPRIDEKY.ORG
QUEER KENTUCKY

MEETING SPACES
SOCIAL EVENTS
LEARNING PROGRAMS
HARM REDUCTION KITS
AND MUCH MORE!

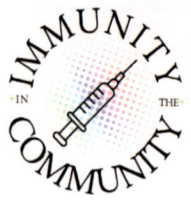

IMMUNITY IN THE COMMUNITY

VACCINE CLINICS
COMING SOON

1324 S. THIRD STREET LOUISVILLE, KY 40203 | 502-498-4298 | INFO@LOUPRIDEKY.ORG

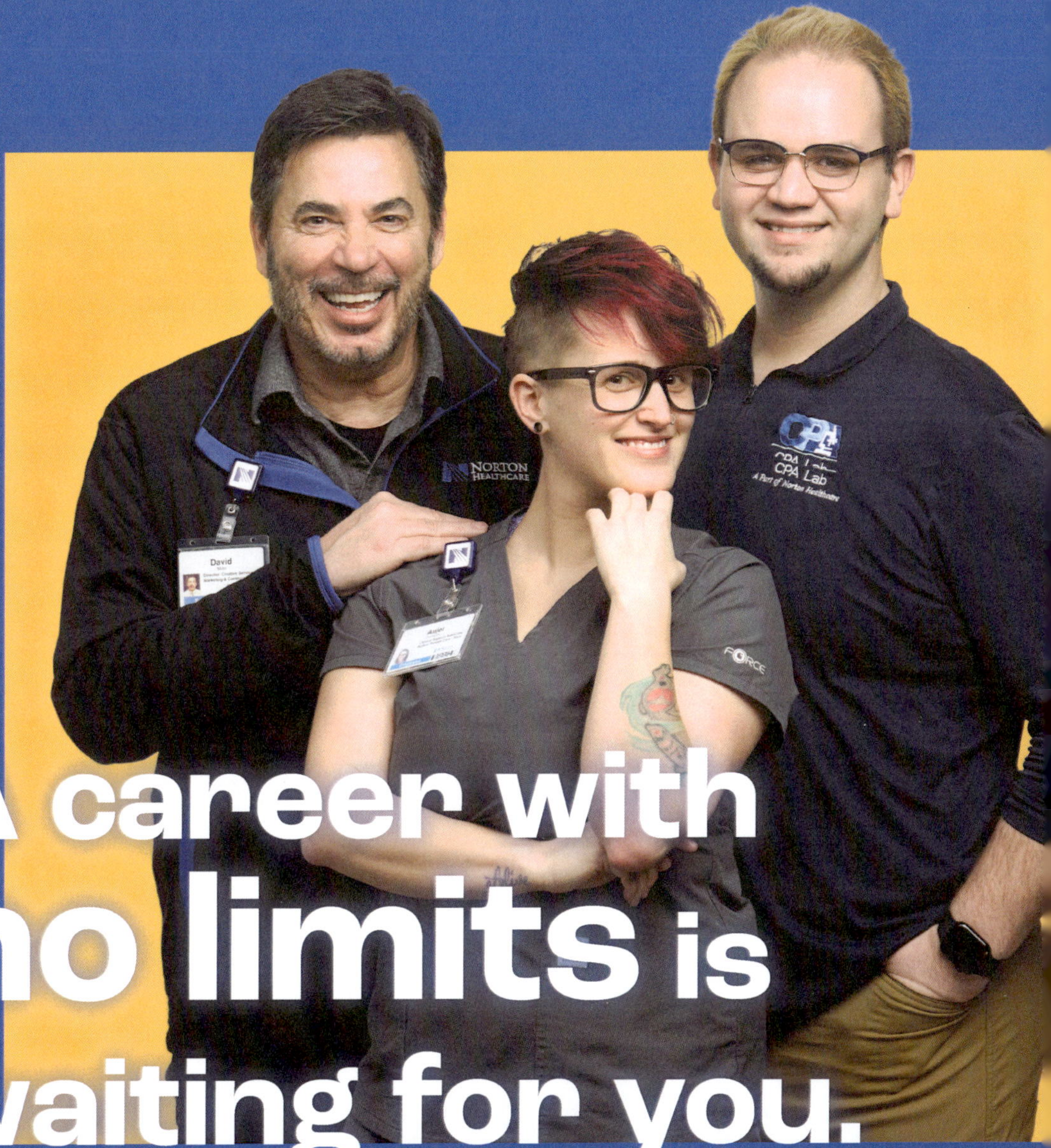

A career with no limits is waiting for you.

Norton Healthcare is unlike any health care system in our region. We're innovators and strategic thinkers. We're researchers, leaders and compassionate caregivers. We're a team — no matter your role or location.

 Scan the **QR code** to discover a career with no limits. You can also email **recruitment@nortonhealthcare.org** or call **(800) 833-7975** to speak with a recruiter.

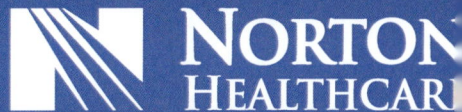

EOE, including disability/vets

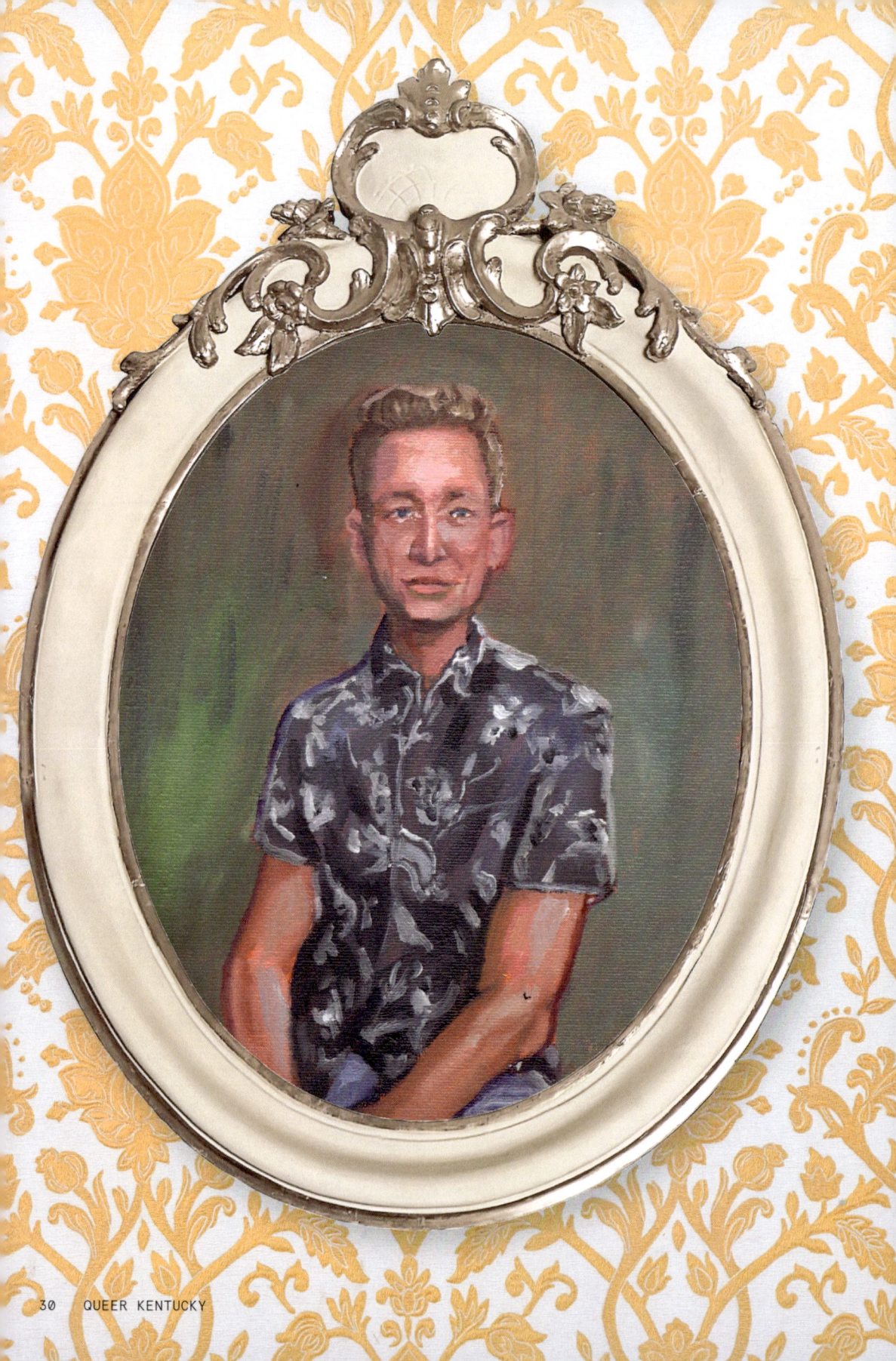

Silas House

LEXINGTON/FAYETTE COUNTY

he/him

Use one Queer slang word to describe Kentucky!

Slang word: Fabulachian (This was coined by two students of mine at Berea College, Sam Gleaves and Ethan Hamblin, in my Appalachian Cultures class, and I think it really captures the spirit of a lot of rural LGBTQ+ Kentuckians.)

How did you activate and organize your community?

I worked with other community members for a couple years to try to get a Fairness Ordinance passed in Berea. We faced huge opposition and harassment for trying to get the ordinance passed and it failed but the visibility of the LGBTQ+ population in the area increased because of this. In response to the ordinance failing I wrote the play This is My Heart for You that was performed to sold out crowds in Berea (and later in Louisville, Pikeville, Morehead, and other places).

We had talkbacks every night to create a better dialogue between the LGBTQ+ community, our allies, and even those who are opposed to our equality. I have also written about these issues for an international audience in publications like Time, The Atlantic, The New York Times, and others. I think I am most proud of trying to expand notions of what it means to be an LGBTQ+ person in a rural place in my own creative work, especially in my novel "Southernmost," my novel "Lark Ascending," and in several short stories that all focus on the Queer experience in Kentucky. Too often the LGBTQ+ experience is limited to two tropes in popular media: being miserable and dying or being the party people/best friends. Our lives are more complex than that, and I want to show us in our multitudes.

In the last 25 years, what is one moment that gave you hope for Kentucky's fight in equality?

When Governor Andy Beshear was elected to a second term as governor. The way we vote is a reflection of our values. Too often Kentucky votes in anti-LGBTQ+ politicians but Governor Beshear not only talks the talk of allyship, he also walks the walk.

What do you think is next for Kentucky in the fight for Equality?

We have to organize as LGBTQ+ people to let the legislators know that we're tired of their anti-LGBTQ+ rhetoric and legislation, both of which are endangering people's lives and freedoms. We have to work together and be more visible. I take real issue with gatekeepers in the state who want to downplay the bigotry that so often occurs here (and is visible in the way the state votes) just so they can keep grants and such rolling in. I think denying the bigotry does a lot of damage. If you love a place you must criticize it and hold it accountable to make it better.

What are Kentucky's greatest strengths when it comes to the fight for Queer equality?

Grassroots organizations. The people are the power. On one hand I hate that the people who are the most impacted by the bigotry are the ones who are having to do the hard work. We have to be out there on the front lines. But on the other hand I am so proud of how we refuse to be silenced.

proudly designed by BRACKISH *a branding studio*

www.brackishcreative.com

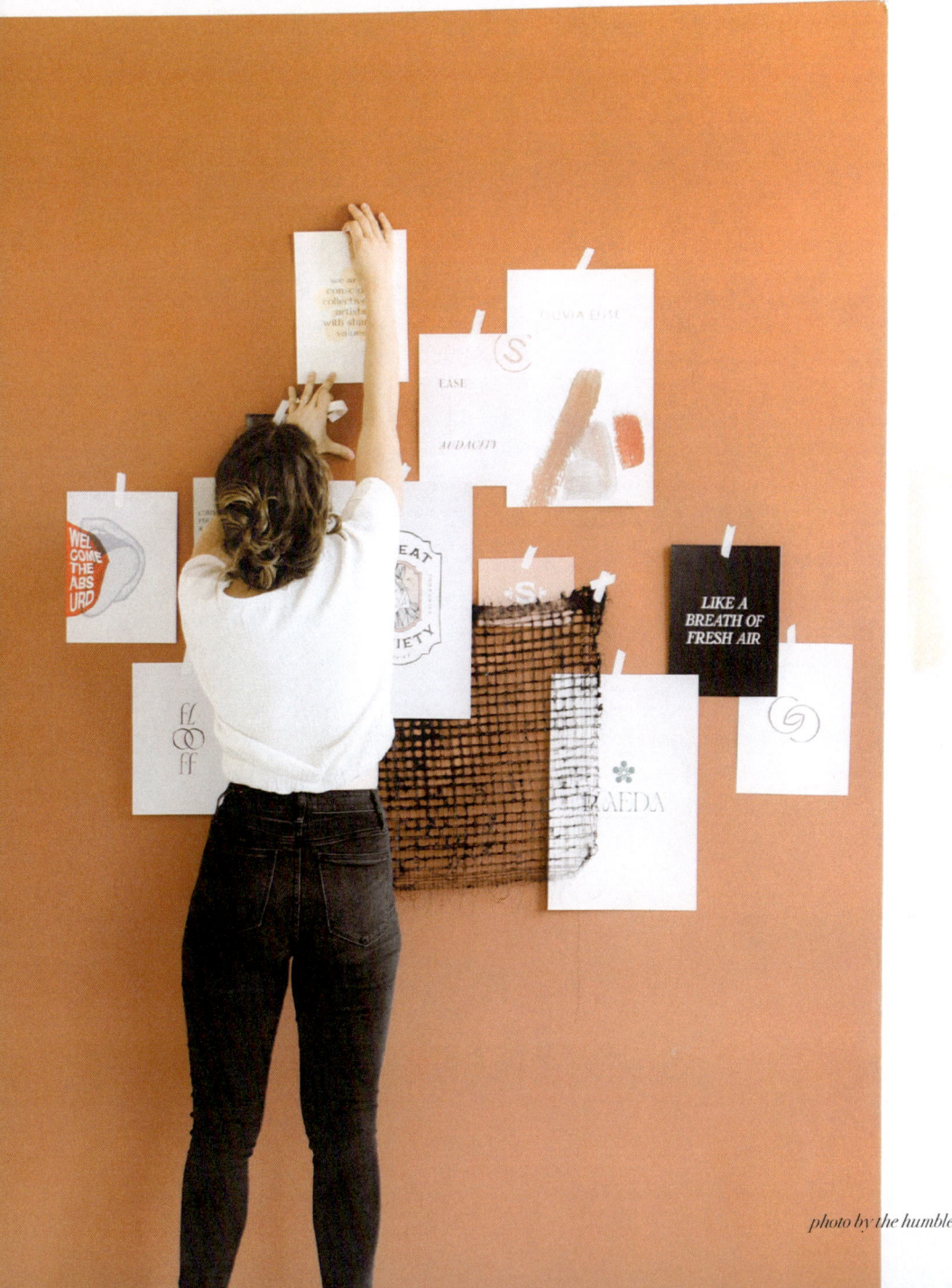

photo by the humble lion

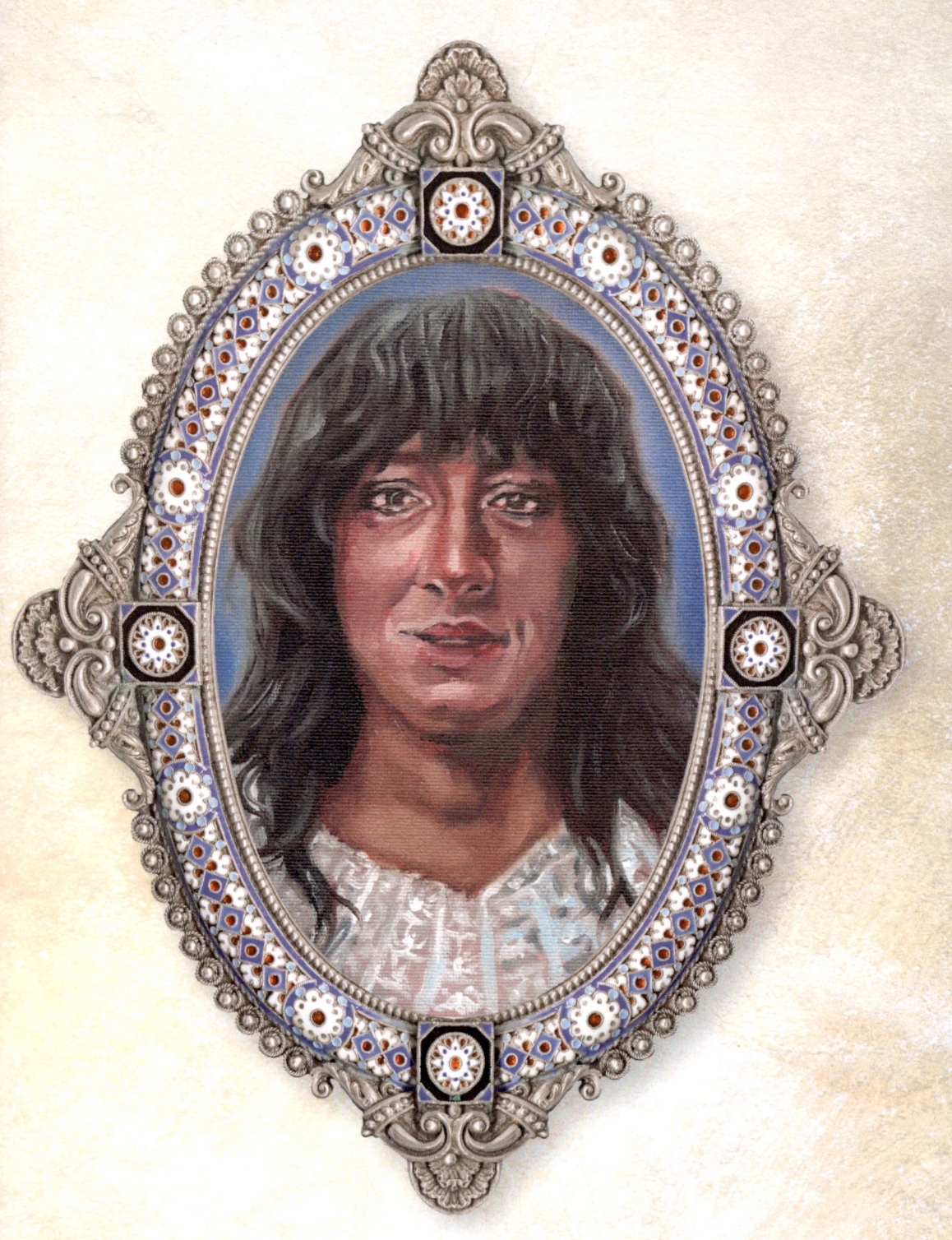

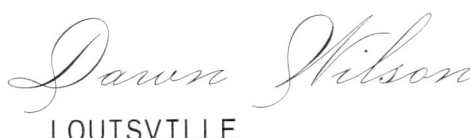
Dawn Wilson
LOUISVILLE
she/her

Use one Queer slang word to describe Kentucky!

Slay

How did you activate and organize your community for equality?

Being present for the community. Using my skills as the Commission's Education Chairperson, responsible to facilitate communications with the community at large in an effort to establish dialogues around the disconnects that exist currently in the educational system dealing with access and diversity. Organizing quarterly dialogue with the Jefferson County School Board, developing a partnership to create an environment that will foster learning at a higher level, engaging parents, educating teachers and advocating for all students especially for our youth and the LGBTQ+ community at large regardless of race, creed or color.

In the last 25 years, what is one moment that gave you hope for Kentucky's fight in equality?

After the merger we were able to combine the city and county Fairness Ordinances into one entity with power to protect everyone.

What do you think is next for Kentucky in the fight for Equality?

Let's start with reinstating abortion rights and restoring the right of parents to decide medical treatment of gender affirming care for their child.

What are Kentucky's greatest strengths when it comes to the fight for Queer equality?

Our tenacity and our resilience. We never give up.

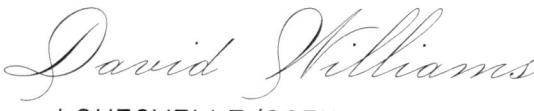

David Williams
LOUISVILLE/SOIN
he/him

Use one Queer slang word to describe Kentucky!

Swish

How did you activate and organize your community for equality?

Founded the Williams-Nichols Collection at the University of Louisville. Have worked for the community in many capacities, including as editor of The Letter, board member of Community Health Trust, and general overall volunteer activity.

In the last 25 years, what is one moment that gave you hope for Kentucky's fight in equality?

When the Fairness ordinances were passed in Louisville and Lexington in 1999.

What do you think is next for Kentucky in the fight for Equality?

Full recognition and protection of transgenders under the law.

What are Kentucky's greatest strengths when it comes to the fight for Queer equality?

The refusal of the community to shrink away when the going gets tough. Sometimes we have had to retreat a little, but that was only temporary.

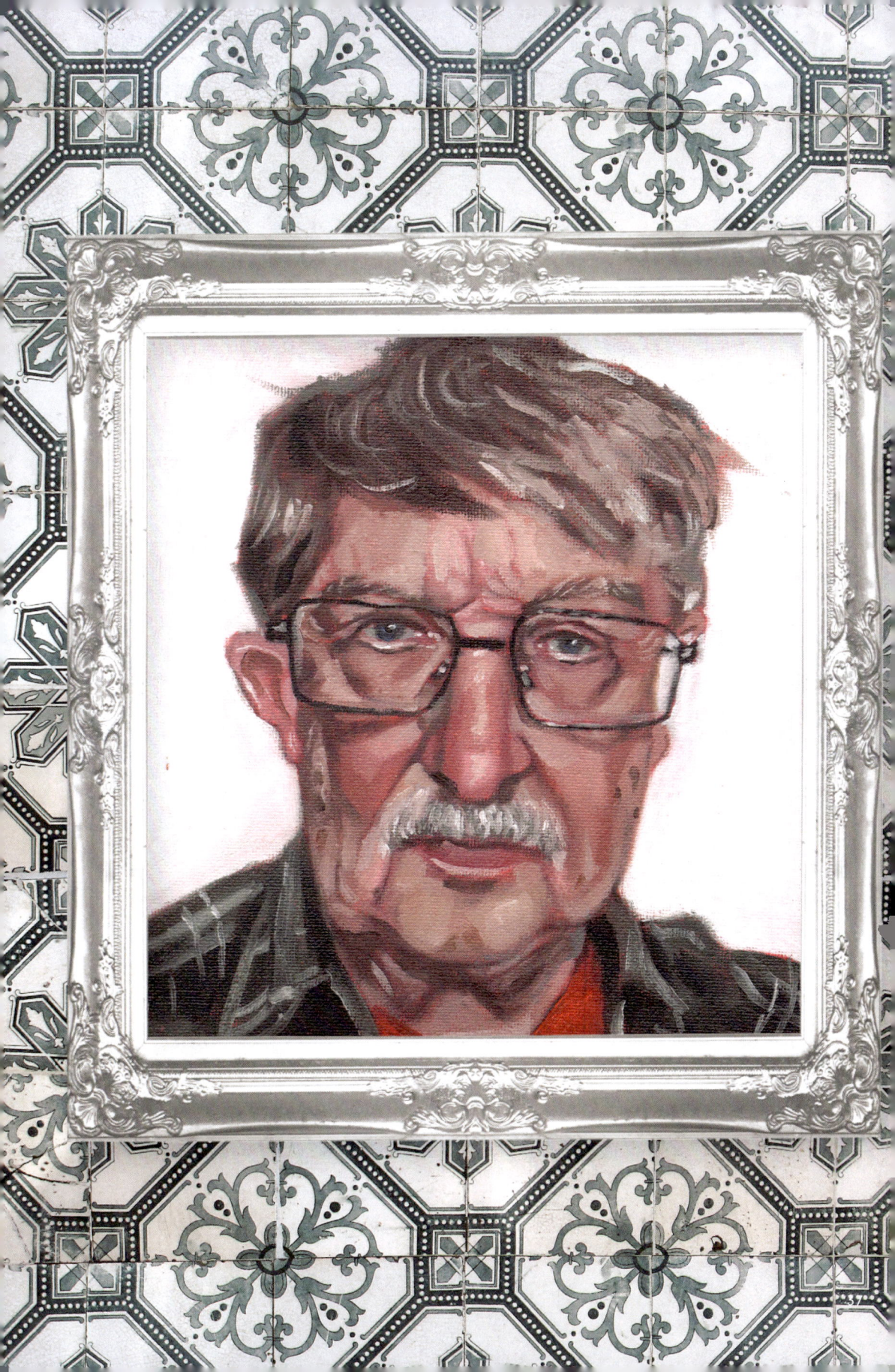

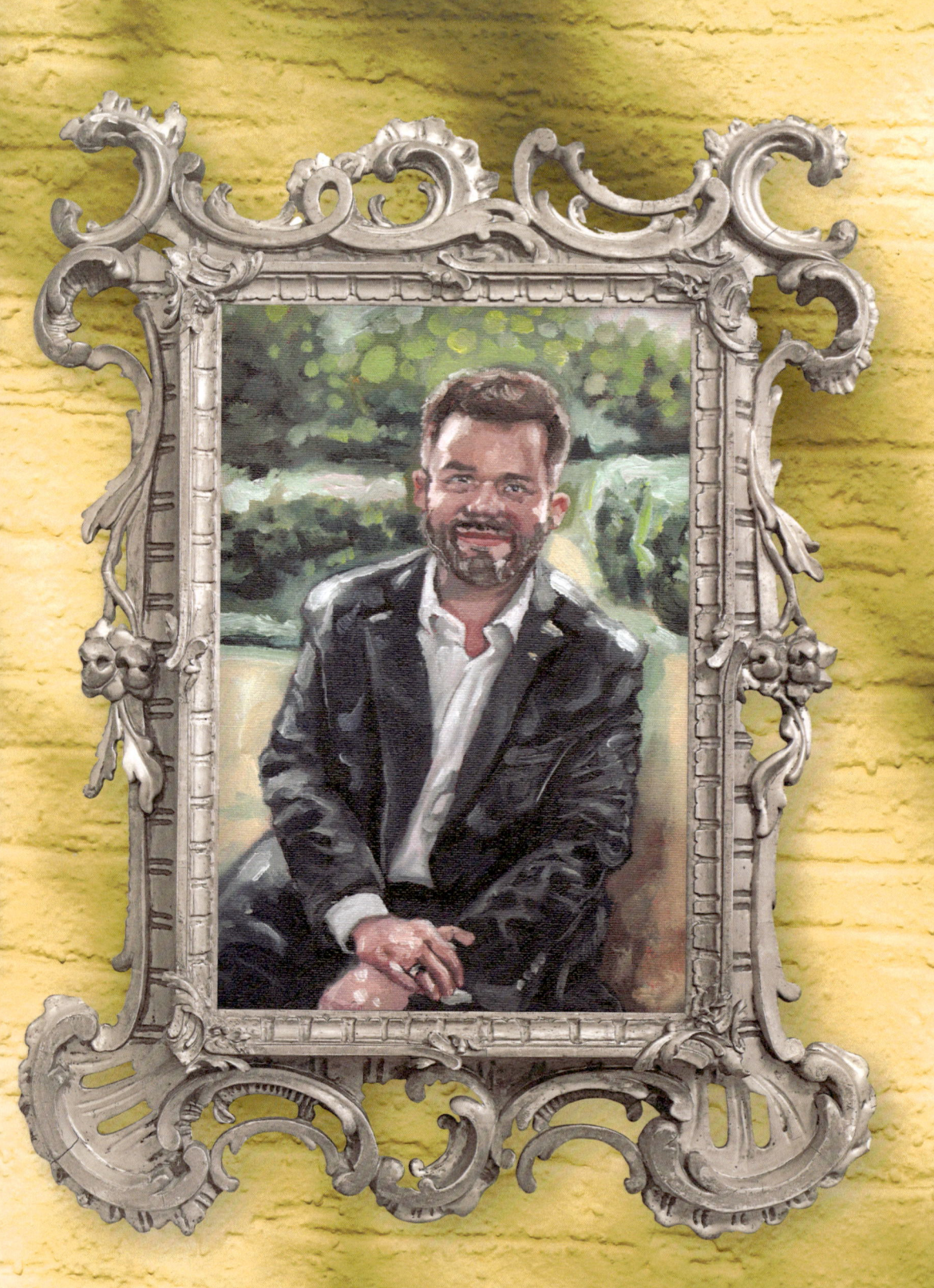

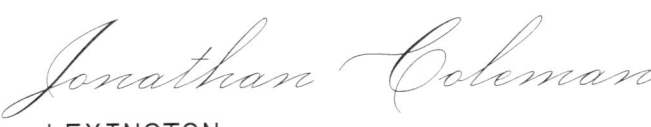

LEXINGTON

he/him

Use one Queer slang word to describe Kentucky!

Verse! The LGBTQ+ community of Kentucky encompasses every walk of life in our Commonwealth. We are drawn from a wide array of social classes, races, ethnicities, religions, abilities, and geographic regions. Nevertheless, we are united in a common Queer experience.

How did you activate and organize your community for equality?

By sharing stories. Kentucky's LGBTQ+ community is one of the brightest threads in the tapestry of our Commonwealth, and our history reflects that richness, offering inspiration, reflection, and hope for change. As we fight our present battles, it's important to know we stand on the shoulders of giants, that we're not the first, and that we've never been alone.

In the last 25 years, what is one moment that gave you hope for Kentucky's fight in equality?

I was running errands on Main Street in Lexington, when I noticed two girls, probably high schoolers, walking past the state's first historic marker commemorating Kentucky's LGBTQ+ history, which the community had installed just about a year earlier. The girls stopped and read it. As they walked away, they clasped their hands together, and continued, hand-in-hand, down Main Street. I knew then that we were going to be alright.

What are Kentucky's greatest strengths when it comes to the fight for Queer equality?

That's easy: Kentuckians. Our people have always been our greatest strength. The ingenuity, sense of fairness, and bravery demonstrated by so many Queer Kentuckians are consistent attributes that this historian knows will not be changing anytime soon.

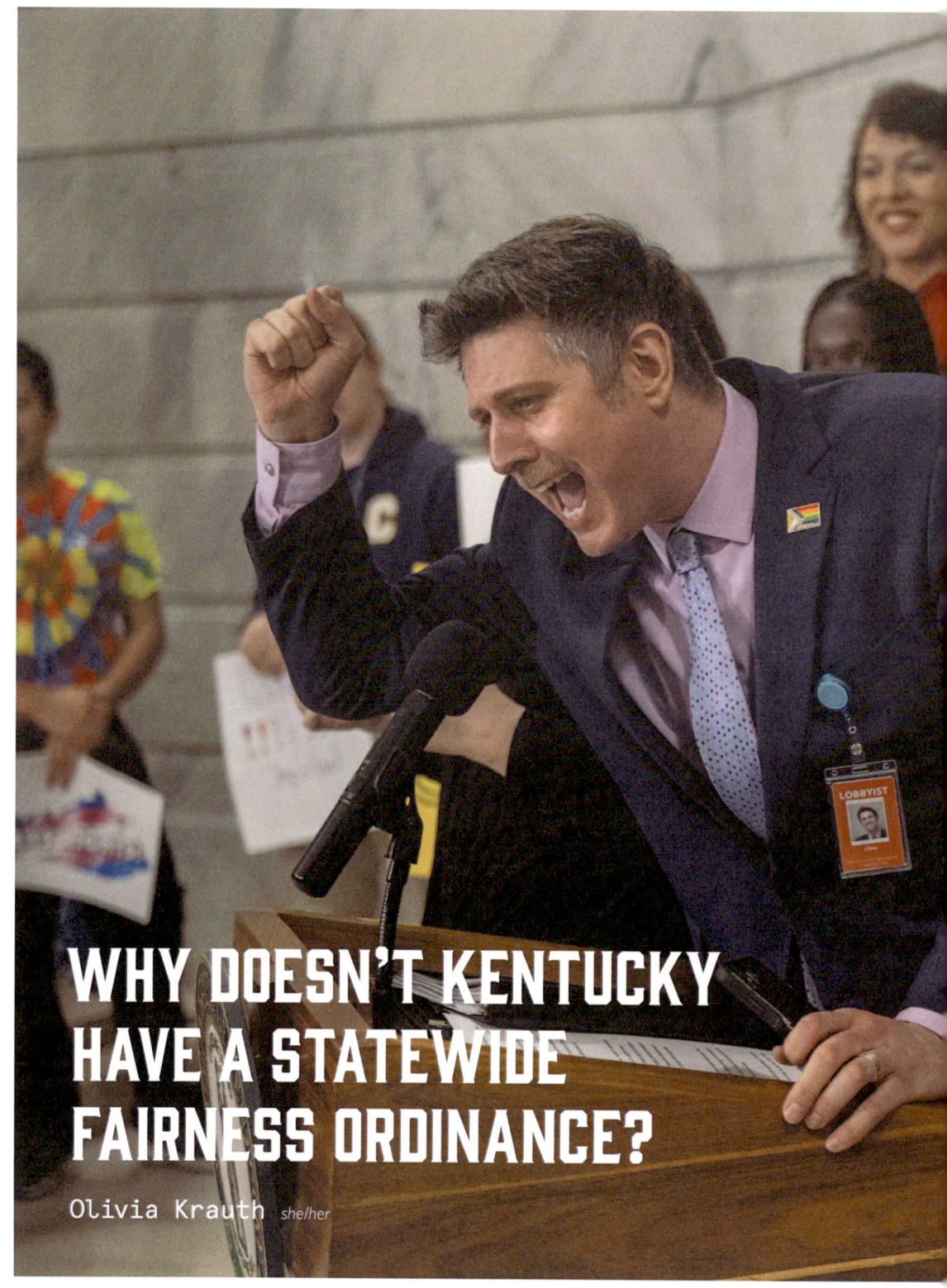

WHY DOESN'T KENTUCKY HAVE A STATEWIDE FAIRNESS ORDINANCE?

Olivia Krauth *she/her*

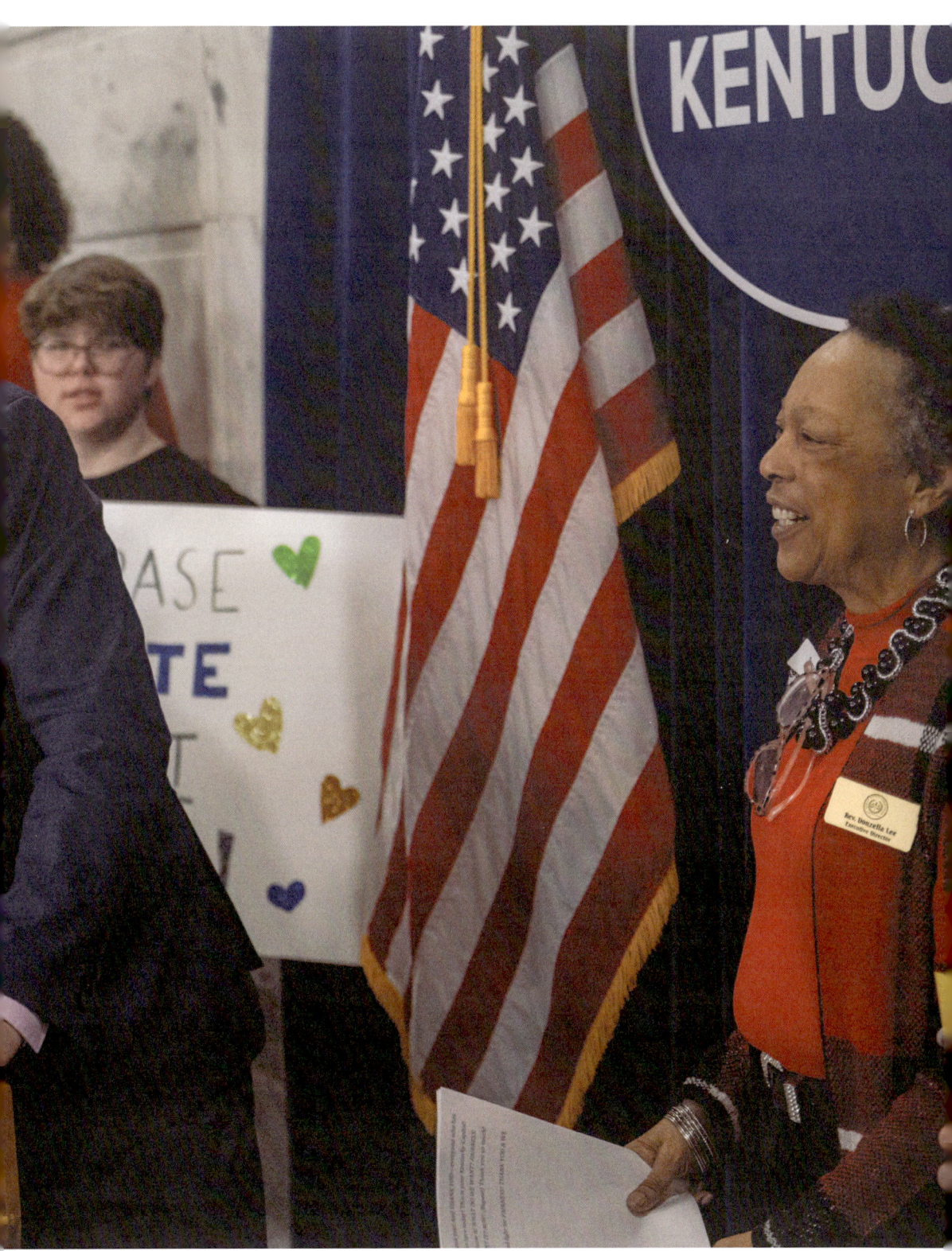

I'm not going to bury the lede, so I'm going to hold your hand while I say something y'all probably already know: Kentucky doesn't have a statewide fairness ordinance.

Around 22 states plus Washington, D.C. have such ordinances in some capacity. Kentucky is not one of them.

Plenty of other states — Kentucky included — have counties or cities with local fairness policies. But, even with two dozen localities in Kentucky enacting their own fairness ordinances, less than one-third of Kentuckians live in areas not protected by such policies.

But it isn't because state lawmakers — well, at least some state lawmakers — haven't been trying. Since Kentucky's 2000 legislative session, nearly 50 bills have been filed to enact some form of statewide fairness.

Obviously, those efforts haven't been successful. Why is that?

NEARLY 25 YEARS OF LEGISLATIVE EFFORTS

Some sort of statewide fairness legislation has been filed in Frankfort nearly every year since 2000.

And since 2003 (again, not counting the pesky 2007 situation), such legislation has been filed in both the House and Senate. At times, House Democrats have tried their chances at filing two similar bills in the same year.

But those legislative pushes have failed. Let me be clear — when I say "failed," I don't mean the bill got a vote or two and just fizzled out. There was nothing to fizzle out. Outside of a few instances, these bills rarely got even a committee assignment when it wasn't required. None of them got a vote, according to legislative records.

Now, it's not uncommon for bills to be filed and not go anywhere in Frankfort. That's actually the reality of most bills that get filed any given legislative session.

But a recent string of high-profile anti-LGBTQ+ pushes from the GOP, coupled with the GOP's sheer dominance over Democrats in the state

Capitol and their focus on leaving things to local governments rather than "big" governments such as the state, can help explain exactly why a statewide fairness ordinance hasn't happened.

THE POWER OF PARTY (OR NOT)

Let's start with the numbers. Democrats — who typically sponsor such legislation — make up less than one-fourth of all seats in the House and Senate. Republicans — who have, on rare occasions, cosponsored such legislation — have a supermajority.

Republicans have repeatedly prioritized anti-LGBTQ+ measures in recent sessions. Keeping trans girls and women out of girls and women's sports. Multiple efforts aimed at limiting drag queens (FYI: this one failed — twice). Banning gender-affirming health care for minors, even if their parents and doctors agree there is a better path. Allowing teachers to misgender their own students if they'd like.

And that means that even though Democratic Gov. Andy Beshear has prided himself on his LGBTQ+ record while in office, pro-LGBTQ+ legislation simply does not make it to his desk.

But, a quick history lesson: Republicans haven't always been completely in charge of the legislature like they are now.

After the 2000 election, 59.4% of the seats in Kentucky's legislature — there are 138 of them — were owned by Democrats and the remaining 40.6% were Republicans.

Now, Democrats make up just 19.6% of those seats while Republicans have 80.4%. And a Democrat has been in the governor's mansion 17 out of the last 25 years, too.

Even though in several situations since 2000, fairness legislation was filed and backed by Democrats in a Democrat-led chamber with a Democratic governor, it still never budged.

"It is far past time for Kentucky to have a statewide fairness law, and we and others in our caucus will never stop trying to make this a reality," Democratic Reps. Keturah Herron and Lisa Willner — both of whom have

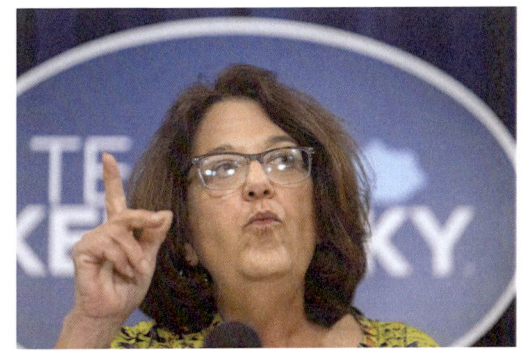

sponsored statewide fairness legislation — said in a joint statement. "Whom you love shouldn't dictate where you can live and work."

WITHOUT STATEWIDE ORDINANCE, EFFORTS MUST BE LOCAL

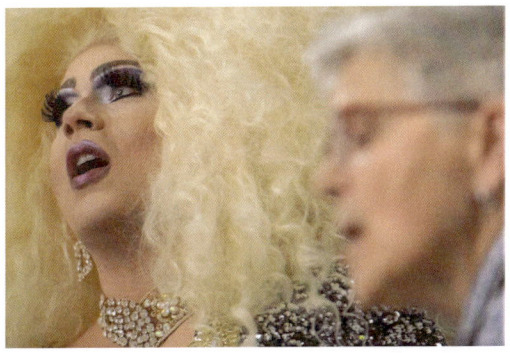

But, the duo continued, "Many of our House and Senate colleagues continue to believe that this issue is better left up to local communities, much like laws governing alcohol sales and public tobacco use."

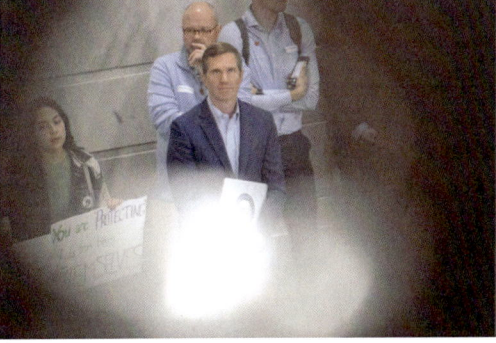

On top of prioritizing anti-LGBTQ+ bills over statewide fairness, many Republicans also generally believe in the concept of small government. Basically, they'd rather leave some decisions up to local communities and their citizens and elected officials, rather than dictate things from a state level.

Now, there are plenty of instances where Republicans overlooked that particular ideal in favor of a more large government approach, but there is a silver lining when it comes to fairness ordinances.

Lack of state action means room for local action, whether that's at the county or city level. Kentucky has 24 local fairness ordinances, though Chris Hartman, the leader of the Fairness Campaign, said that may shift soon.

But just because local fairness ordinances are allowed right now, doesn't mean that could last forever.

Herron and Willner said "with the legislature more and more inclined to preempt local ordinances," pointing to a recent state removal of some cities' housing ordinances, "there is growing fear that fairness protections now in place for half of Kentuckians could be next."

One way to act? Vote, they said.

"If we want a more inclusive, fair, and just commonwealth," Herron and Willner said, "we must elect leaders who believe in that for everyone, no matter their gender or sexual orientation/preference."

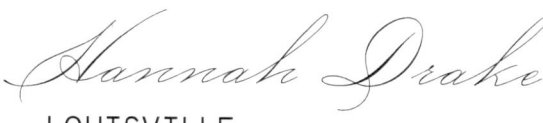

LOUISVILLE

she/her

What do you think is next for Kentucky in the fight for Equality?

As Beyoncé said in her song American Requiem "Nothing really ends. For things to stay the same they have to change again." The fight for equality and fairness for LGBTQ+ people will not end because the discrimination will just shape shift to something else. I do not believe that LGBTQ+ people can ever grow complacent because hatred never takes a day off it will also think about what it can morph into and look new but it is the same old hate. I also believe it is a MUST that if you are LGBTQ+ do not wait until the bell tolls for you specifically. Wherever you see injustice it is also your fight because hate and discrimination does not ever stop with one group of people. It will soon be knocking at your door. If you see Black people fighting for justice, stand up! If you see women fight for women's rights, stand up! If you see injustice, stand up! Only by standing together do we empower ourselves and the next generation.

What are Kentucky's greatest strengths when it comes to the fight for Queer equality?

The People are the biggest strength and asset of the LGBTQ+ community. The People are the ones who will demand equality, fairness and justice. The People are the ones that will carry the message, that will march in the streets, that will stand up and say this is wrong. The People are the ones that will require this state to change. We are only as strong as The People.

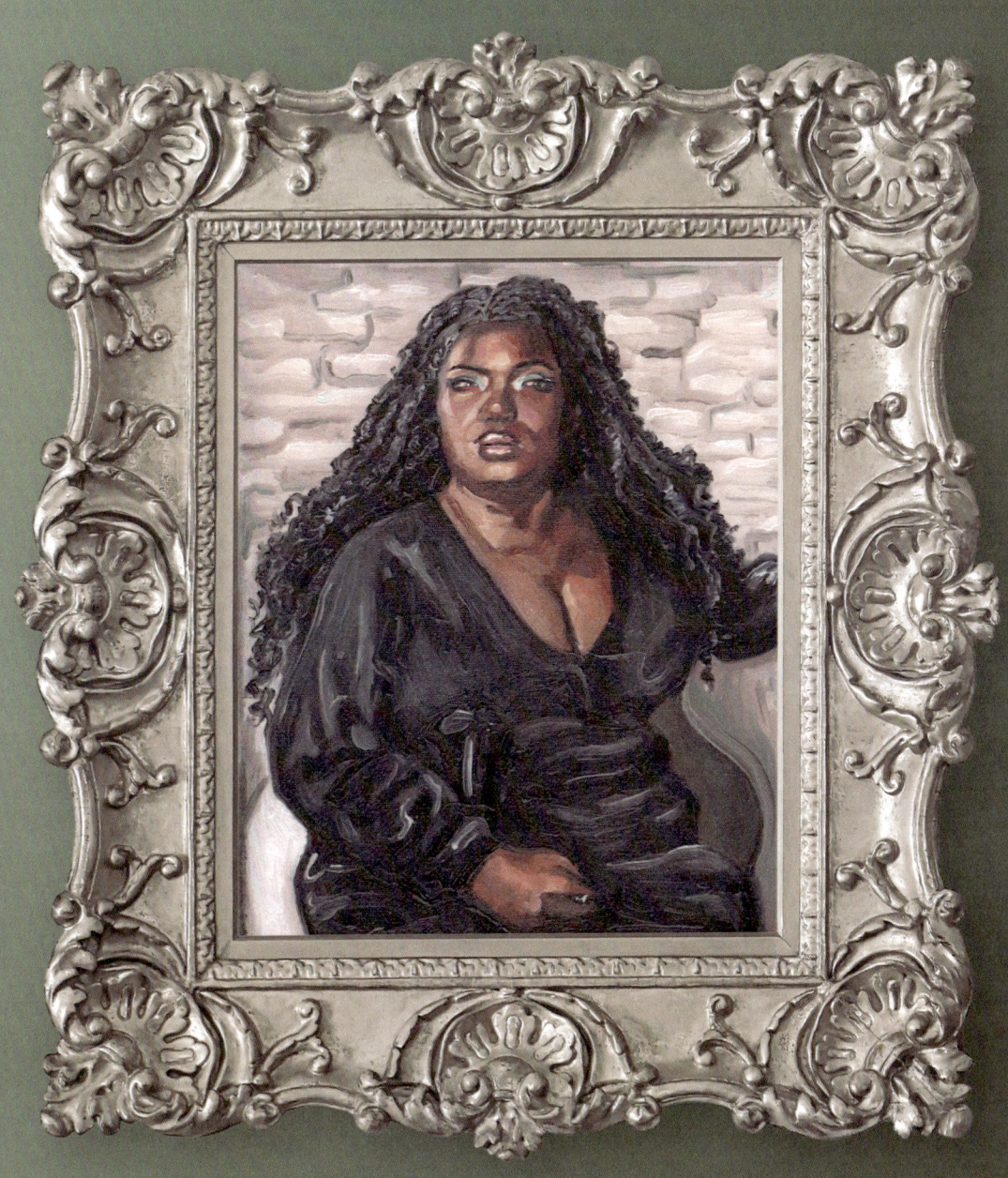

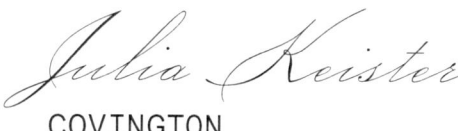

COVINGTON

she/they

Use one Queer slang word to describe Kentucky!

"queer-pas-gay"

How did you activate and organize your community for equality?

By creating spaces and experiences that fully embody and empower Queerness. Queer not only in the limiting terms of identity, but Queer because it is a place of community, of celebrating difference, of acceptance, of experimenting, of learning and of truly being yourself.

In the last 25 years, what is one moment that gave you hope for Kentucky's fight in equality?

About 5 years ago, when the parent of a Trans Girl Scout asked if her daughter could set up a table to sell cookies at our shop. An immediate feeling of, "We are all going to be okay." rushed over me.

Who is one other LGBTQ+ Kentucky leader that you admire and why?

Non-living = Bell Hooks, because of her fearless and unwavering dedication to justice, as well as her general badassery.

Living = Each and every Queer Kentucky kid, and all of their friends. The youth are the real rainbow warriors fighting the most important, and most difficult, battles daily. They are the ones who will ensure that the future is QAF.

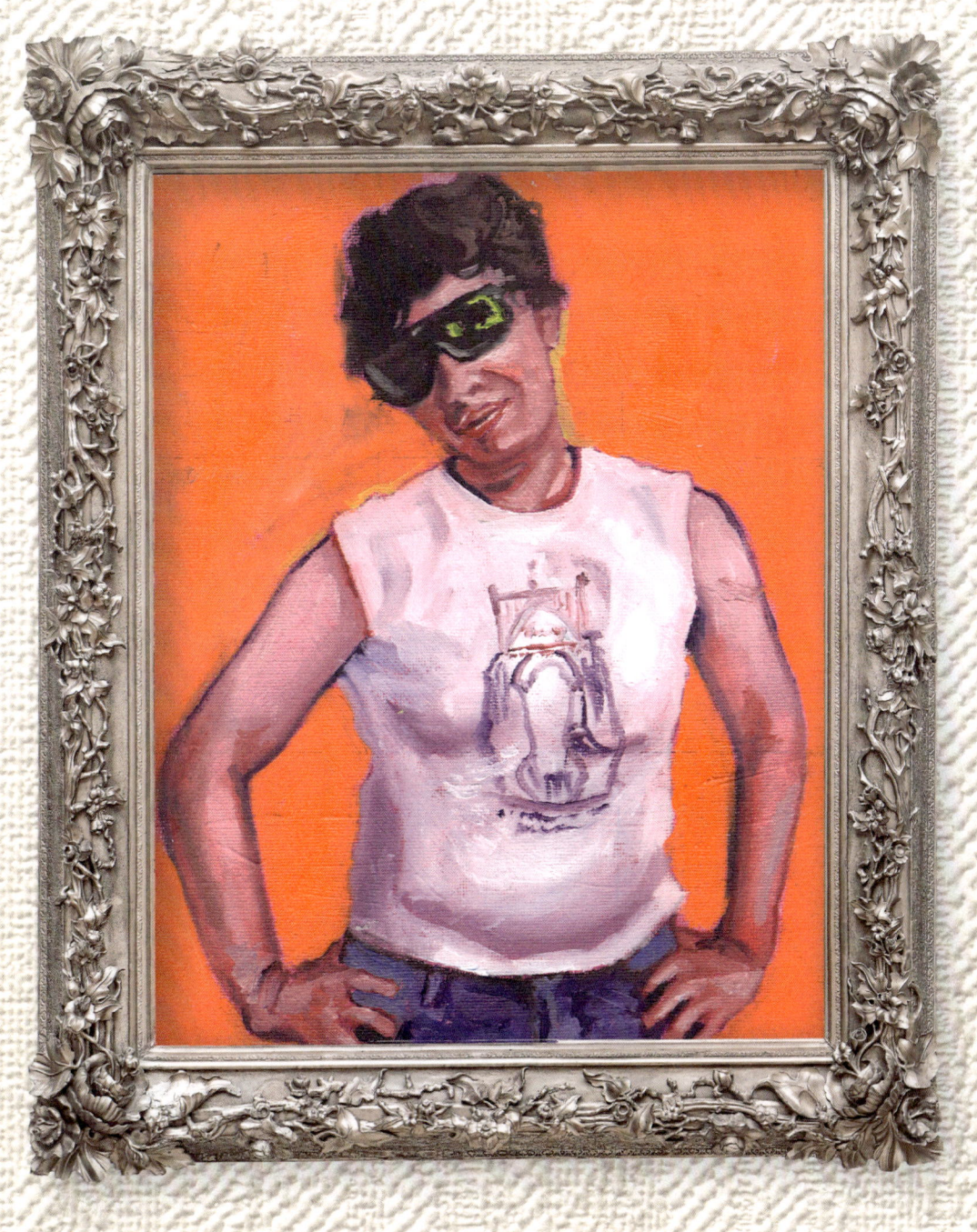

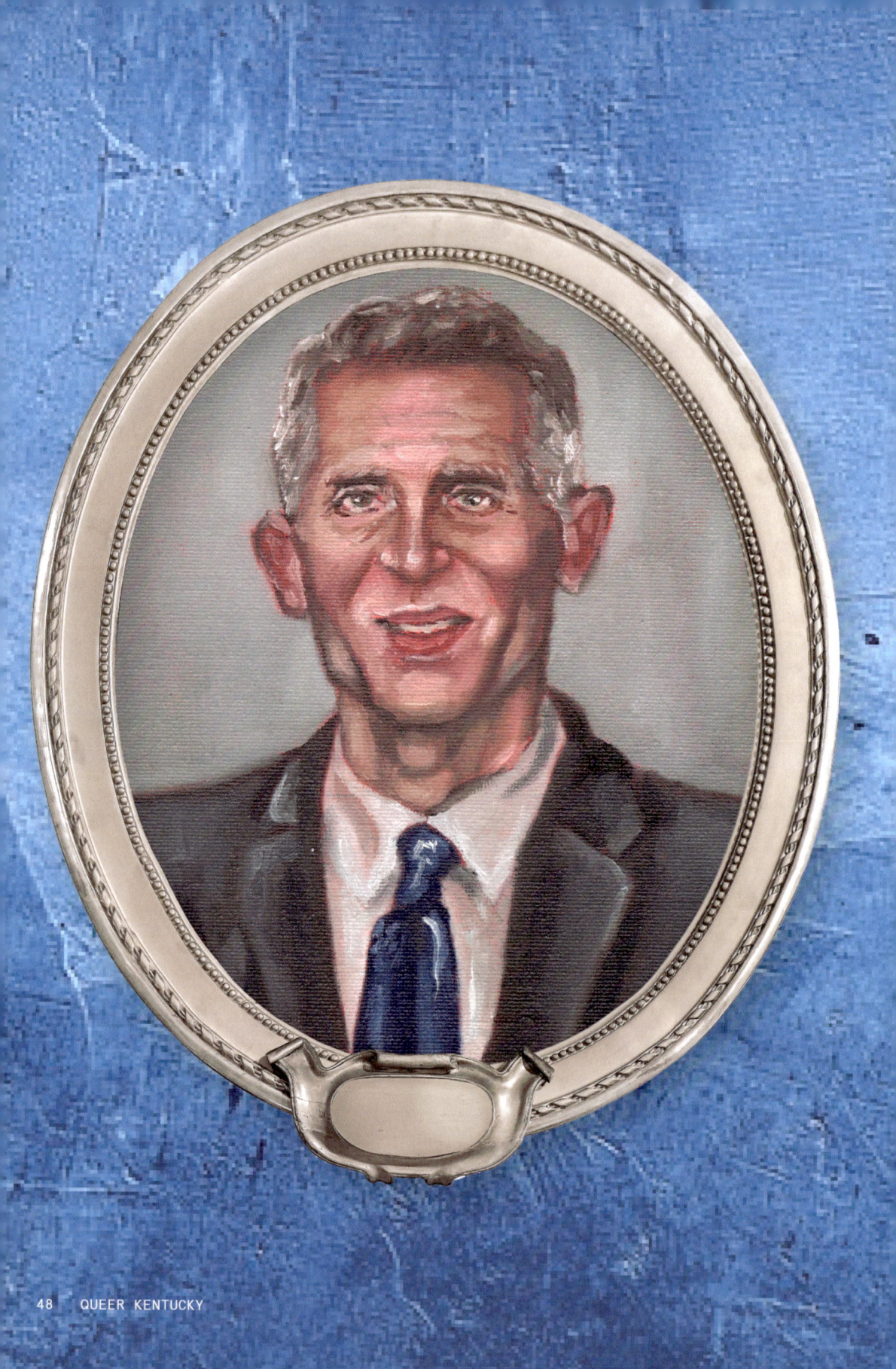

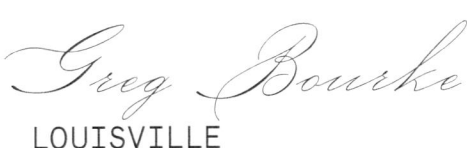

Greg Bourke
LOUISVILLE
he/him

Use one Queer slang word to describe Kentucky!

Queer. It seems cliche but as someone who has been out since 1976, I remember how hateful and condemning this term used to be for anyone who didn't fit the cis hetero normative criteria. It was a horrible and demeaning insult that was used frequently. Now people don't bat an eye when they hear this term in Kentucky, the script has been flipped, it is perceived generally as a positive. In one term, for me this symbolizes how far Kentucky has come.

How did you activate and organize your community for equality?

After being removed in 2012 from my position as a scoutmaster for our son's boy scout troop, I launched a campaign to pressure the Boy Scouts of America to revise its membership policies and eliminate its ban on gay scouts, as well as, gay and lesbian adult scout leaders. Working with Scouts for Equality, GLAAD and change.org, these policies were successfully revised in 2014 and 2015 making scouting now much for inclusive LGBTQ+ people.

In the last 25 years, what is one moment that gave you hope for Kentucky's fight in equality?

June 26, 2015 when the Supreme Court ruled that marriage equality was a right all Americans deserved under the law. This ruling brought such joy and relief to the LGBTQ+ community and was also heralded by our countless allies as a turning point in the long fight for LGBTQ+ equality and inclusion. Obviously, other challenges still remain, and new ones have emerged since then, but that was a moment of great hope and accomplishment for so many.

What do you think is next for Kentucky in the fight for Equality?

Trans rights have been under attack for the last several years in Kentucky, particularly by our state legislature. We all need to rally behind the defense of those impacted by this hateful and unnecessary targeting of the trans community.

What are Kentucky's greatest strengths when it comes to the fight for Queer equality?

Kentucky's free-spirited people who believe in the freedom and equality we are all guaranteed under the Constitution, Kentucky people, for the most part, believe that all have the right to be their full and true selves, and the government should not be dictating how we can identify and live our lives. One remarkable aspect of Kentucky is how broadly marriage equality is now accepted by Kentuckians, after it was so widely rejected by 75% of voters in passing a constitutional same-sex marriage ban in just 2004.

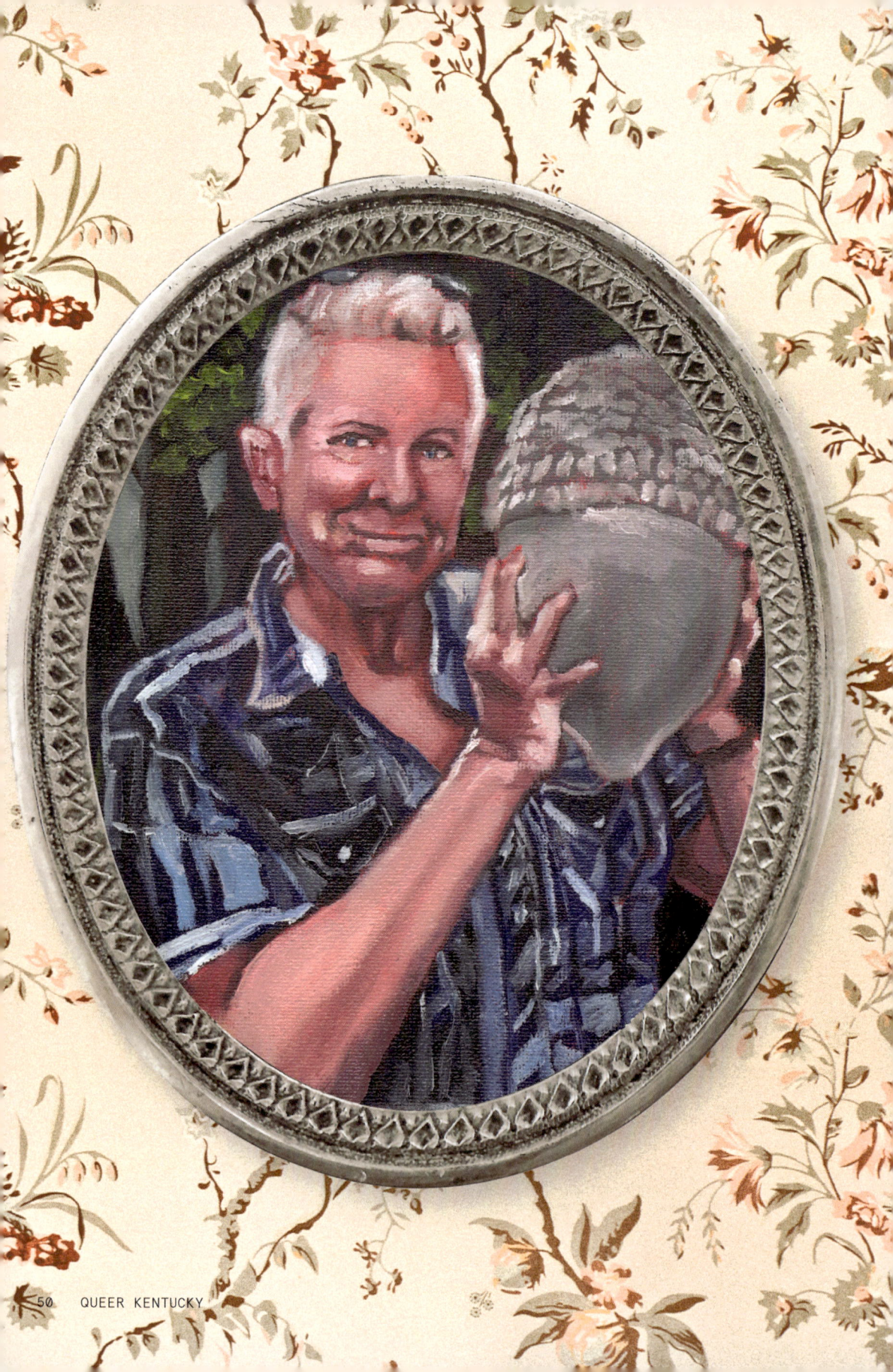

Laura Petri (AKA RESIN REBEL)

PADUCAH

she

Use one Queer slang word to describe Kentucky!

Paducaaah is Leztopiaaah! Who knew?

How did you activate and organize your community for equality?

I have spent my life as an activist…a feminist…and an organizer.

In 1993, I was selected to serve on the inaugural statewide steering committee for the Kentucky Fairness Alliance.

In the mid-1990's I published a local LGBTQ+ newsletter called "A Common Thread" which announced networking opportunities, community organizing events and LGBTQ+ social events in and around Paducah.

In the 1990's I was a recipient of a Kentucky Foundation for Women grant for "Grassroots Women Present," and served as site producer for a traveling play about Belinda Ann Mason, a Kentucky writer who contracted the AIDS virus through a transfusion.

I served on the Paducah Pride committee, and was instrumental in helping initiate and organize the very first Paducah Pride events in the 1990's.

Because of my community organizing skills and my passion for LGBTQ+ work (although I do not identify as Christian) I was recruited to serve as a founding board member of the LGBTQ+ friendly Metropolitan Community Church of Paducah.

Serving as a worker at lesbian and women's festivals for over two decades has given me the confidence and vision to plant my "acorns" locally. When the Michigan Womyn's Music Festival ended in 2015, after 40 years of providing a safe space for women, we were tasked to "sprout our acorns" in our home towns to create women's community and events.

In 2016, I sprouted my "acorn," Cinema Systers Film Festival, a four day women's cultural festival in Paducah. In addition to screening lesbian produced films, we have filmmaking workshops, Q&As, LGBTQ+ musicians, comedians, spoken word artists, open mic, karaoke, DJs, dancing, catered parties, networking opportunities, art displays, silent auction and more.

Our nonprofit organization My Syster's Art, Inc., was founded in 2019 to produce Cinema Systers and other events throughout the year which empower women and LGBTQ+ folks.

Lastly, The Art Farm Women's Retreat was established on our 34 acre farm outside Paducah to further our intention of creating safe spaces for women and our LGBTQ+ sisters and brothers. We have hosted many events, and just added an outdoor stage, with plans to host festivals and fundraisers for the causes we care dearly about. (seen on HipCamp and Airbnb).

In the last 25 years, what is one moment that gave you hope for Kentucky's fight in equality?

Formation of Kentucky Fairness Alliance in 1993.

I was honored to serve on that founding KFA Statewide Steering Committee.

More recently...

When Gov. Andy was elected!

What do you think is next for Kentucky in the fight for Equality?

1) Let's start with reinstating abortion rights. Stripping women's bodily autonomy is a wake-up call...a foreshadowing of many more human rights to be violated and/or vacated.

2) Changing the hearts and minds of the MAGA contingent/religious zealots is a huge obstacle to achieving equality. Exposing the general public to stories of LGBTQ+ folks' struggles to live authentically can go a long way toward humanizing us.

3) We must always strive to recognize allies and stand for racial, socio-economic, gender, and all forms of equality. There is strength in numbers.

4) We must flip Kentucky blue to move forward in our quest for equality. GOTV (get out the vote) campaigns are extremely important to our success as a community, a commonwealth and a country. So go vote... and bring 100 friends.

What are Kentucky's greatest strengths when it comes to the fight for Queer equality?

Pockets of Kentucky have a progressive vibe, such as Paducah and Louisville.

I can personally attest the Paducah Convention and Visitors Bureau (CVB) has been a wonderful ally to our international lesbian film festival (Cinema Systers Film Festival).

R.I.P. Mary Hammond, the late CVB Executive Director and an extraordinary friend of our community.

Our local NPR station (WKMS 91.3) at Murray State University has been an ally to Cinema Systers, as well. Acts of inclusivity and support like theirs can go a long way toward the success of LGBTQ+ endeavors, and the normalization of gay people.

The Kentucky Foundation for Women continues to support female artists statewide in projects that are socially impactful.

Brave and dedicated individuals across our Commonwealth who take an active role in civil and political discourse are sheros and heros in our movement to abolish inequality.

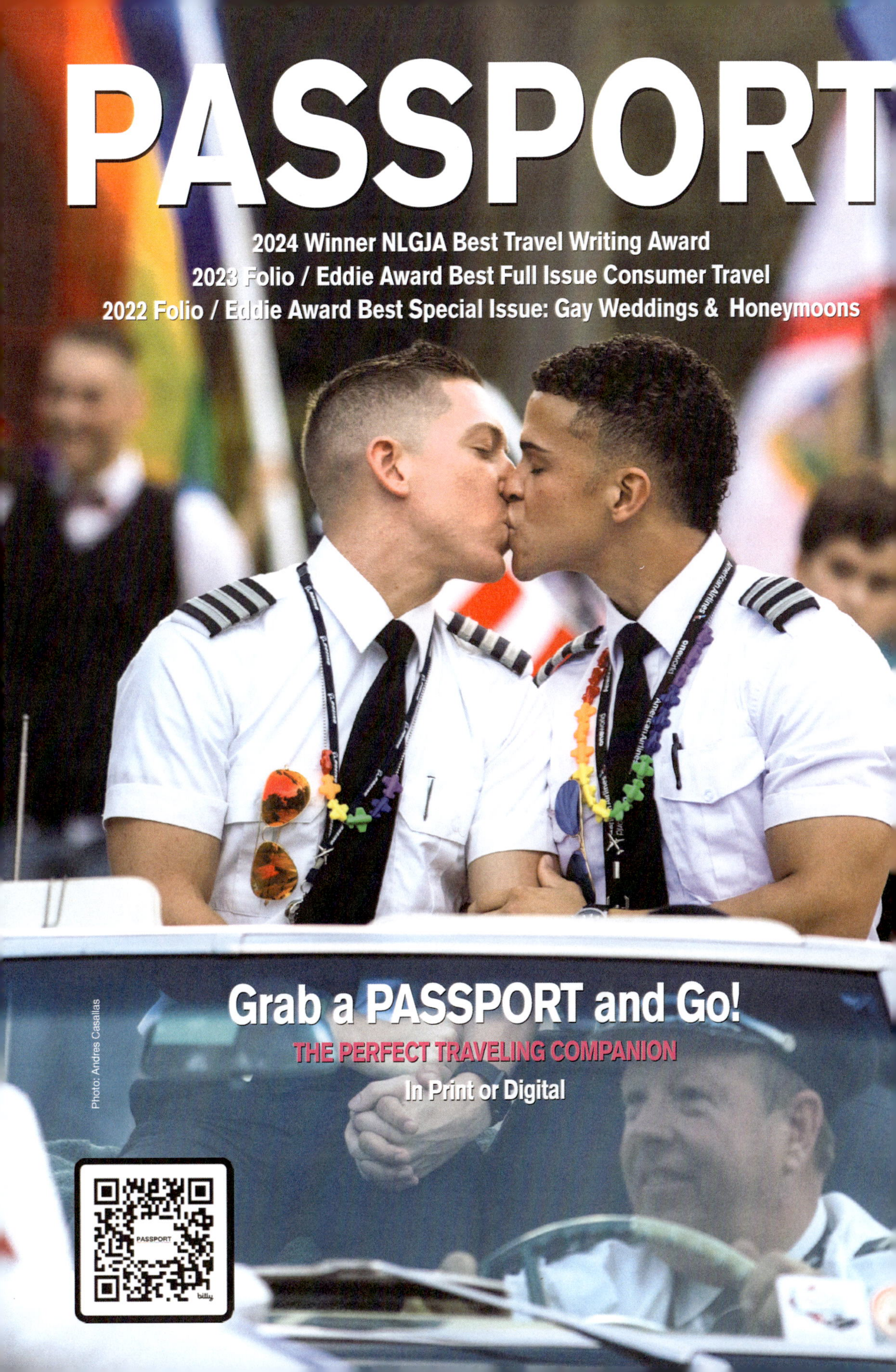

PASSPORT

2024 Winner NLGJA Best Travel Writing Award
2023 Folio / Eddie Award Best Full Issue Consumer Travel
2022 Folio / Eddie Award Best Special Issue: Gay Weddings & Honeymoons

Photo: Andres Casallas

Grab a PASSPORT and Go!
THE PERFECT TRAVELING COMPANION
In Print or Digital

TRAILBLAZER: KENTUCKY'S HIGHEST
RANKING LGBTQ+ POLITICIAN,
Jim Gray

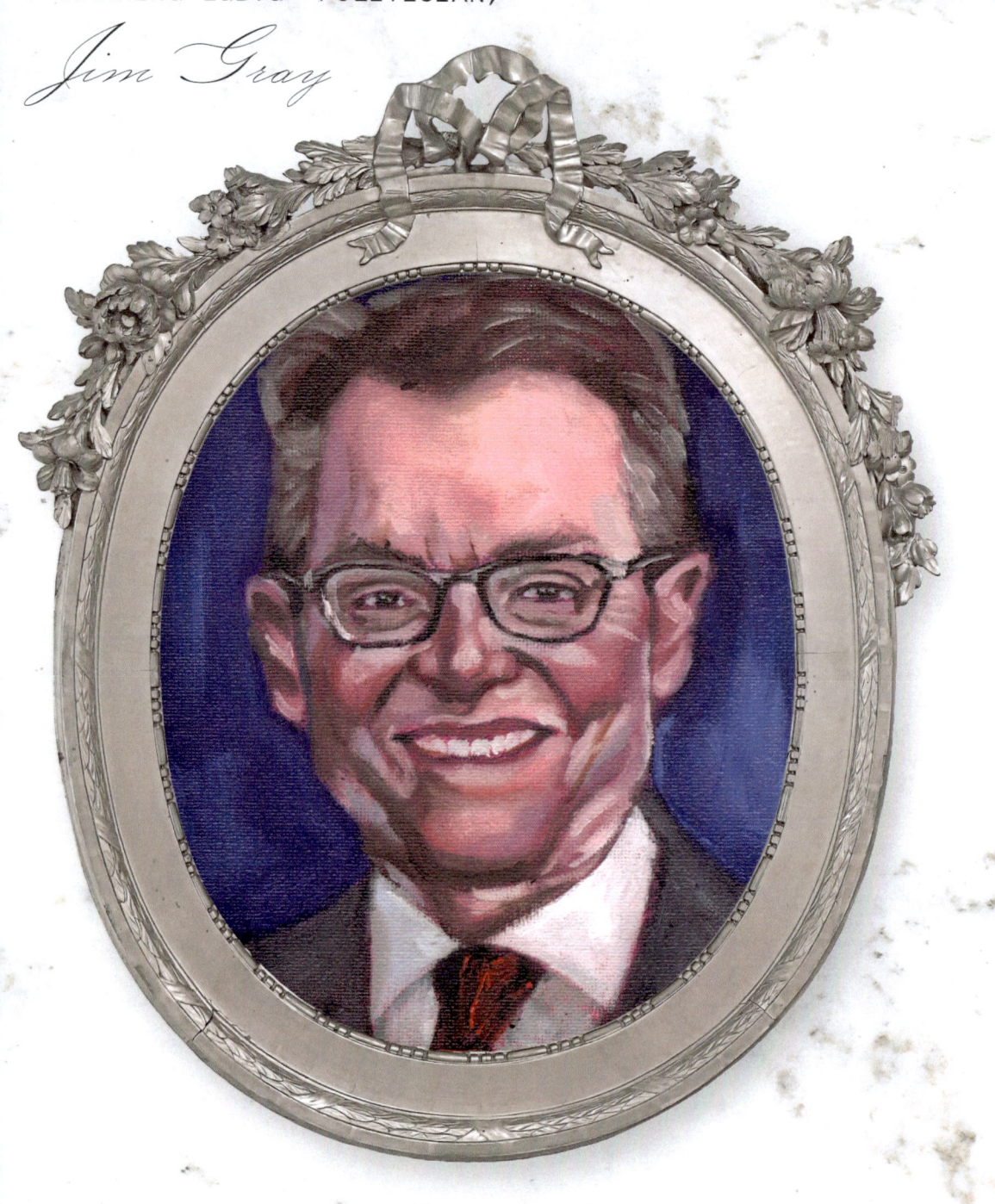

Silas House *he/him*   @silashouse

Jim Gray is sitting beneath a large portrait of him that hangs in the bar of the 21C Hotel in Lexington. In the striking photo collage created by James Robert Southard, there are many nods to his city-altering term as mayor of Lexington from 2011-2019. There's the historic courthouse he had restored, an image of a newspaper story about his decision to relocate Confederate statues from the courthouse's lawn, the remodeled and expanded Rupp Arena and Central Bank Center that has helped to reenergize downtown, and many other allusions to the tremendous impact he had during his eight years in office.

Gray doesn't seem to notice I have purposely chosen this spot to sit. He's just returned from a trip to Japan and South Korea with Governor Andy Beshear, and his sleep schedule has been stunned by jet lag, but he is eager to get back to work. When I tell him I am interviewing him because he's thought of as a hero of fairness by many, he blushes.

"Well, I never think of myself that way," he says, as a good politician would. But the difference with Gray is he's being authentic. Unlike most politicians, one of Gray's foundational traits is his modesty. Those who have known him for years may not even know he is a graduate of Vanderbilt and was a Loeb Fellow in the Harvard College of Design, as he never mentions either fact. When he was 19, he became the second youngest person in history to serve as a delegate to the Democratic National Convention. But he has always been proud that he was the first openly gay mayor in Kentucky. Today, as Kentucky's Secretary of Transportation, he is the highest-ranking LGBTQ+ politician in the Commonwealth.

His counterpart at the federal level is Pete Buttigieg, the nation's first openly gay cabinet member. When Gray first met him years ago, Buttigieg told him he was "a trailblazer." Gray still seems surprised by the compliment, even though it's a word that is often associated with him.

Bernadette Barton is a professor of sociology and gender studies at Morehead State University and one of the founders of Just Fund, an organization dedicated to promoting fairness in the state. She has been grateful for Gray's service. "Alongside the peace and prosperity Lexington enjoyed under Mayor Gray, I especially appreciate that he was a trailblazer for the LGBTQ+ community in the Bible Belt, normalizing sexual diversity and helping evaporate the stigma of the closet," she says.

"I know he'll rebuff this statement, but I'm going to say it anyway: Jim Gray is a history-maker," says Jon Coleman, director of the Faulkner-Morgan LGBTQ+ Archive in Lexington. "The bravery he has shown…as an openly gay man cannot be understated. I know, for me personally, what it meant just to witness him walking in Lexington's parades as both a candidate and as mayor, or entering the inaugural ball with [his partner] Eric by his side. What a proud legacy he has made for himself, and for us."

Gray says one of his proudest achievements as mayor was the controversial move to install rainbow crosswalks in downtown Lexington, near a block that is associated with gay bars and restaurants. He knew he would be attacked, even though no tax dollars were used for the project; it was paid for by a grant from the Bluegrass Community Foundation.

Those rainbows made many LGBTQ+ people feel seen, just as Gray's visibility has. Sometimes the very act of existence as a Queer person is a revolutionary act, and Gray is grateful he has had the opportunity to be in the public eye as a gay person during a time of volatile rhetoric and legislation— and a time in which many politicians still cannot come out. "Sadly, people feel they have to be closeted for many reasons, still, and I was lucky that I had a family that was generally embracing, almost to a person…it took a long while to get to that point," he says. "And there are still ramifications for people who come out, there is still fear and anxiety."

He knows that from experience. When Gray first ran for mayor of Lexington in 2002, he was still closeted. "There were lots of whispers, lots of speculation. I was not at all comfortable declining or denying it, and wouldn't do that, so after that I was determined to not go through that again." He came out later in life, at the age of 53, and in 2016 ran against Rand Paul for the U.S. Senate. On the campaign trail across the entire state, he says he had encounters with a couple of people who were "not violent, but aggressive" about him being openly gay. Meanwhile, the New York Times and other national publications ran pieces about a gay man running for federal office in a red state.

"I put myself to the full test there of going back to my roots and going to communities around the state where I had done work as a businessman, with the full knowledge that I was out and that I was really challenging the cultural norms," he says. Although he lost the race, Gray was buoyed by the way his hometown turned out to support him, and talking about that is the only time he grows a bit emotional during our conversation.

"I'll never forget going to Glasgow on the final day of the campaign and I didn't know if it'd be five or ten people or twenty people, but I sure didn't expect 200," he says. Gray is proud of his rural Kentucky roots, but he struggled with the overwhelming conservative leanings. "As much as I'm attached through family and history and to my hometown, family that grew up there, I wanted to get out of there because of fear, fear that I couldn't be authentic, couldn't live an authentic life," he says.

Gray strongly values his LGBTQ+ community and says he believes that there is "bonding through experiences" as members of marginalized groups. He says that affinity allowed him to better understand the opposition to Lexington's Confederate statues that he was instrumental in getting removed after the group Take Back Cheapside raised the issue. "Arguably it cost me the 2018 congressional race," he says, referring to his primary run against Amy McGrath. "But I felt it was [the right thing], especially after a Black teacher told me, 'How would you like to walk down the street and see a statue to a fellow who had fought to keep your ancestors and your people in slavery celebrated in the most central public space in the town?' That really resonated with me."

These days, Gray serves in the cabinet of Governor Andy Beshear, whom he says is the "most pro-LGBTQ+ governor, ever, in the South." In 2019, Gray and his longtime partner, Eric Orr, were famously the first gay couple to be introduced together at a Kentucky inauguration, and Gray says he's felt the full support of Governor Beshear.

"He's about the golden rule," Gray says of Beshear. "He transparently lives his values and those are Christian values. He translates that faith in an unusually positive and affirming way."

Gray looks back on his early days in politics and hesitantly agrees with me that he's been a part of change. "When I got into politics I… definitely had an aspiration to make a difference…and to be a role model," he says, but that's as far as he will go. Even if he won't brag on himself, many others will, and he has earned a permanent place in Kentucky's fairness and LGBTQ+ history.

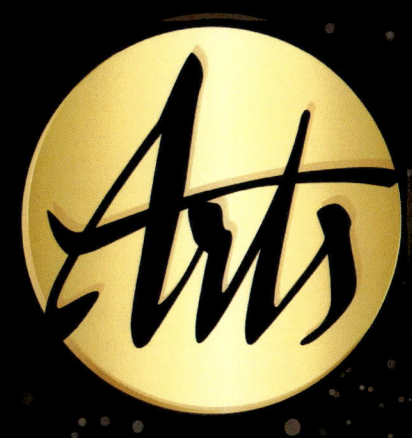

Arts

75 YEARS IN THE CITY OF ARTISTS

CELEBRATE WITH US AT
FUNDFORTHEARTS.ORG

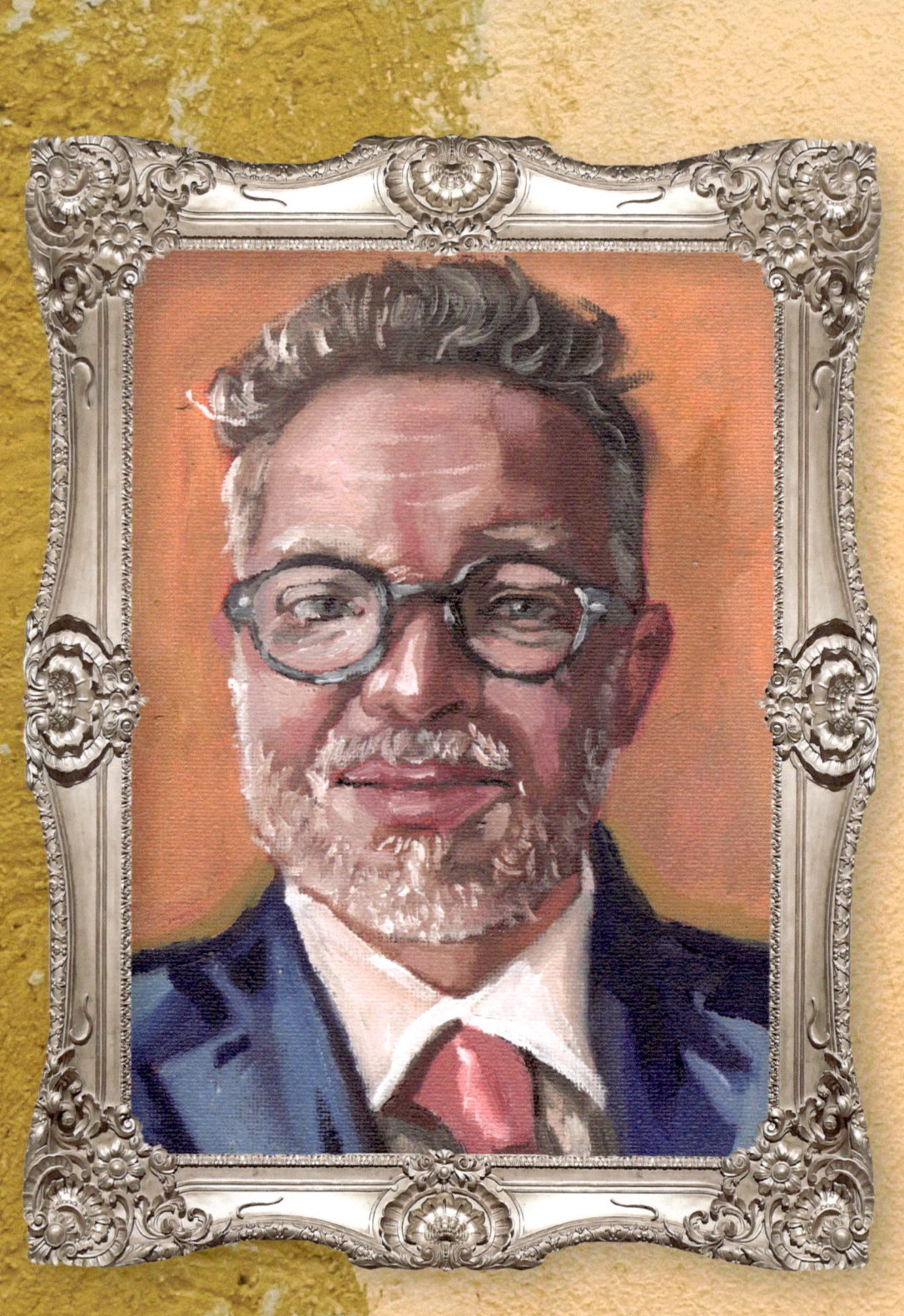

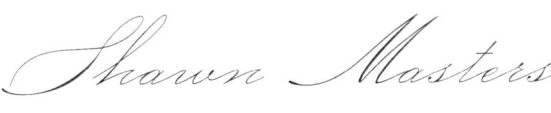

COVINGTON

he/him

Use one Queer slang word to describe Kentucky!

Giddy-up

How did you activate and organize your community for equality?

I've been involved in promoting equality since 2003. That year the city of Covington was one of the first to pass a Fairness Ordinance, and I was a vocal advocate for its passage. Fast forward to 2008, when I ran as the first open-gay candidate for Covington City Commission. I served two terms and was instrumental in proposing, and advocating for passage, domestic partner benefits for Covington city employees.

In the last 25 years, what is one moment that gave you hope for Kentucky's fight in equality?

There isn't one moment, in particular. When I look back on the early 2000s, compared to today, the fundamental change—despite the conservative efforts to curtail our progress—is that the vast majority of the people I know, and especially the younger generation, just don't give a damn about someone's sexual preference. It's refreshing to see their "live and let live" attitude. I do believe, however, that continued education of gay issues, the prominence of gay/gay-friendly media/tv icons has really assisted in our fight for equality even among those we might not have initially thought were allies. Our government tries to divide, but the heart and soul of true Americans want to unite.

What do you think is next for Kentucky in the fight for Equality?

Unfortunately, very little if we continue to elect those who, time and time again, advocate for reclassifying us as second class citizens through legislation and language.

What are Kentucky's greatest strengths when it comes to the fight for Queer equality?

Our greatest strength is what has always been Kentucky's greatest strength: Its people!

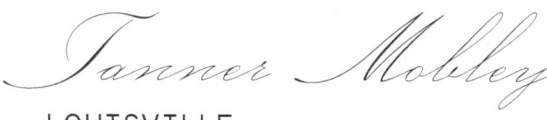

Tanner Mobley

LOUISVILLE

he/him

Use one Queer slang word to describe Kentucky!

Kentucky's fluid—people claim we're a Red stronghold, but we're actually very purple and swing both ways.

How did you activate and organize your community for equality?

I kicked off a grassroots movement in Kentucky to ban conversion therapy, educating hundreds of thousands of Kentuckians on its dangers. Together with an amazing team of organizers, we mobilized thousands to push for statewide legislation to protect minors and played a pivotal role in passing bans in Covington, Lexington, and Louisville. In 2021, we achieved one of the highest Republican co-sponsorship rates for a pro-LGBTQ+ bill in history. Today, at The Trevor Project, I'm dedicated to expanding protections for LGBTQ+ young people nationwide. After eight years of dedicated advocacy, I, along with a coalition of Kentucky organizations, successfully secured an executive order signed by Governor Beshear to protect minors from conversion therapy.

What do you think is next for Kentucky in the fight for Equality?

Kentucky is one of the most disenfranchised states in the country, with many people too busy trying to survive to organize for change. In my experience traveling across the state, Kentucky is full of kind-hearted, resilient folks who care deeply for our families and neighbors. I sense a reckoning on the horizon—people are fed up with the status-quo and ready for change. By uniting Queer Kentuckians and all communities that have been screwed over by the system, I believe we can one day transform Kentucky and make significant strides toward equality.

Who is one other LGBTQ+ Kentucky leader do you admire and why?

I deeply admire my friend Zach Meiners, for his courage and unwavering advocacy to protect LGBTQ+ young people conversion therapy. His tireless efforts in pushing for legislative protections, along with his impactful documentary 'Conversion' highlighting survivor stories, have undoubtedly saved lives. Zach's advocacy is a true testament to the power of storytelling and effecting change.

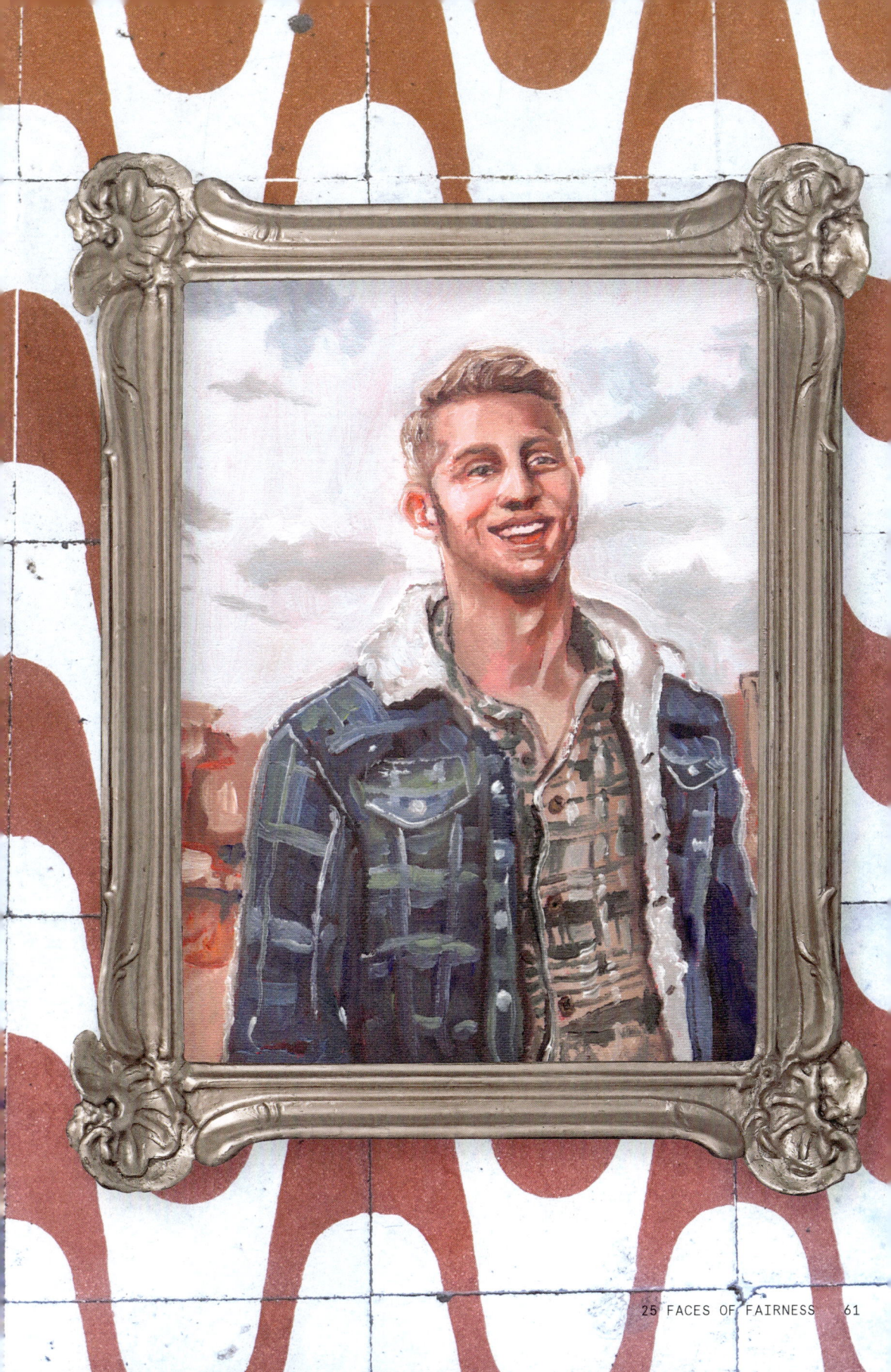

25 FACES OF FAIRNESS 61

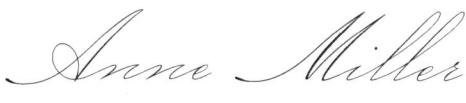

LOUISVILLE

she/they

Use one Queer slang word to describe Kentucky!

I have absolutely no idea! Not Queer specific, but y'all is a personal favorite.

How did you activate and organize your community for equality?

I think the Fairness Ordinance in the late 1990's in Louisville made incredible strides, though on a personal level, I tend to feel the most hope when interacting with young folks. The upcoming generation is fearless, and incredible.

In the last 25 years, what is one moment that gave you hope for Kentucky's fight in equality?

I think we likely have a lot to do in maintaining the rights that have already been established, in addition to working towards greater protections for LGBTQ+ youth.

What do you think is next for Kentucky in the fight for Equality?

We have wonderful grassroots organizations, and a culture of peer support that is really special. I think the diversity within the Queer diaspora of Kentucky is also a huge strength, especially when efforts towards equality are pooled. It makes us difficult to ignore, or dismiss.

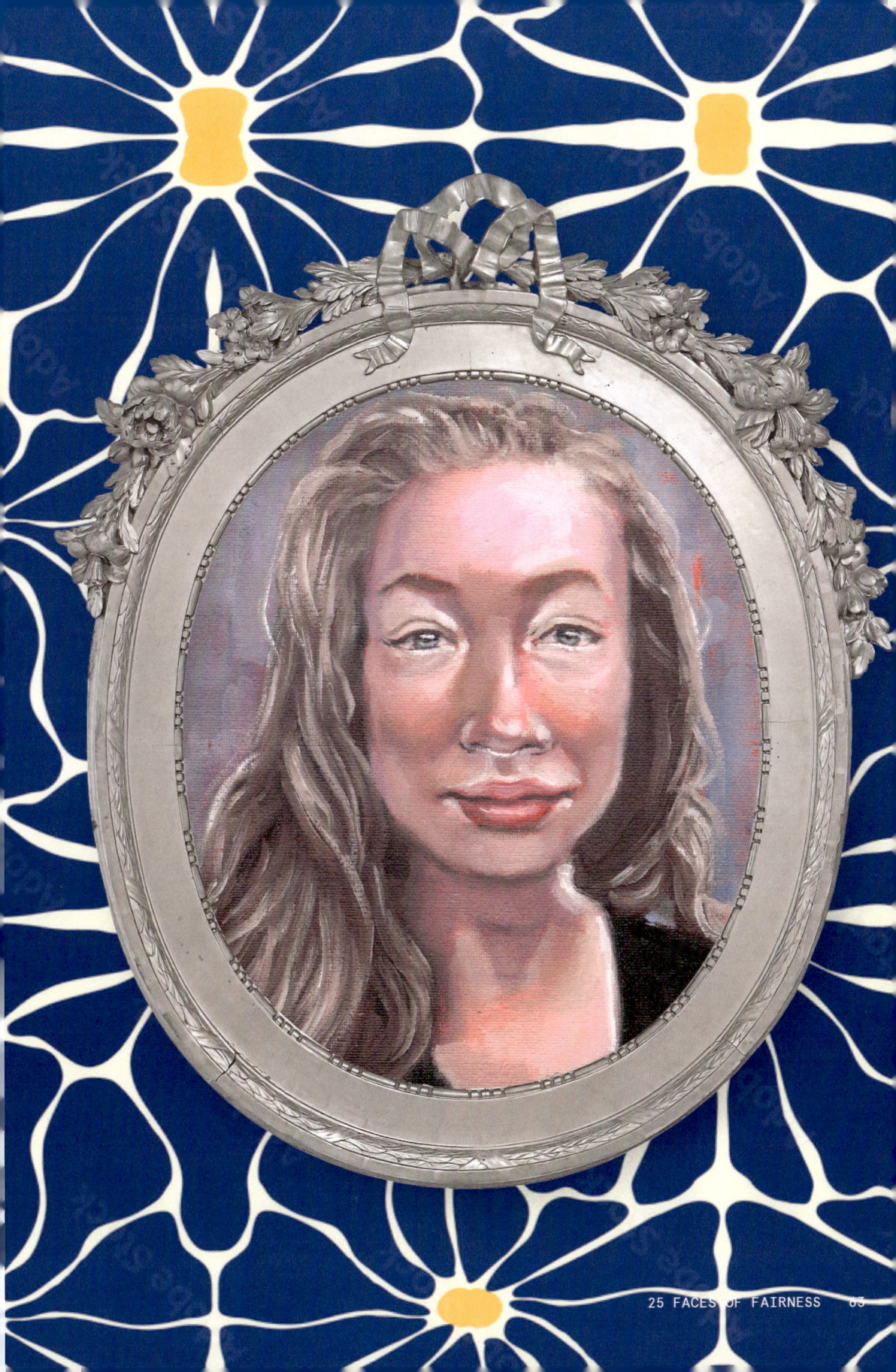

RELIABLY QUEER, SAFE, AND GOOD:
Day's Espresso and Coffee

Belle Townsend *she/they* *@belletownsendky*

@daysespressoandcoffee

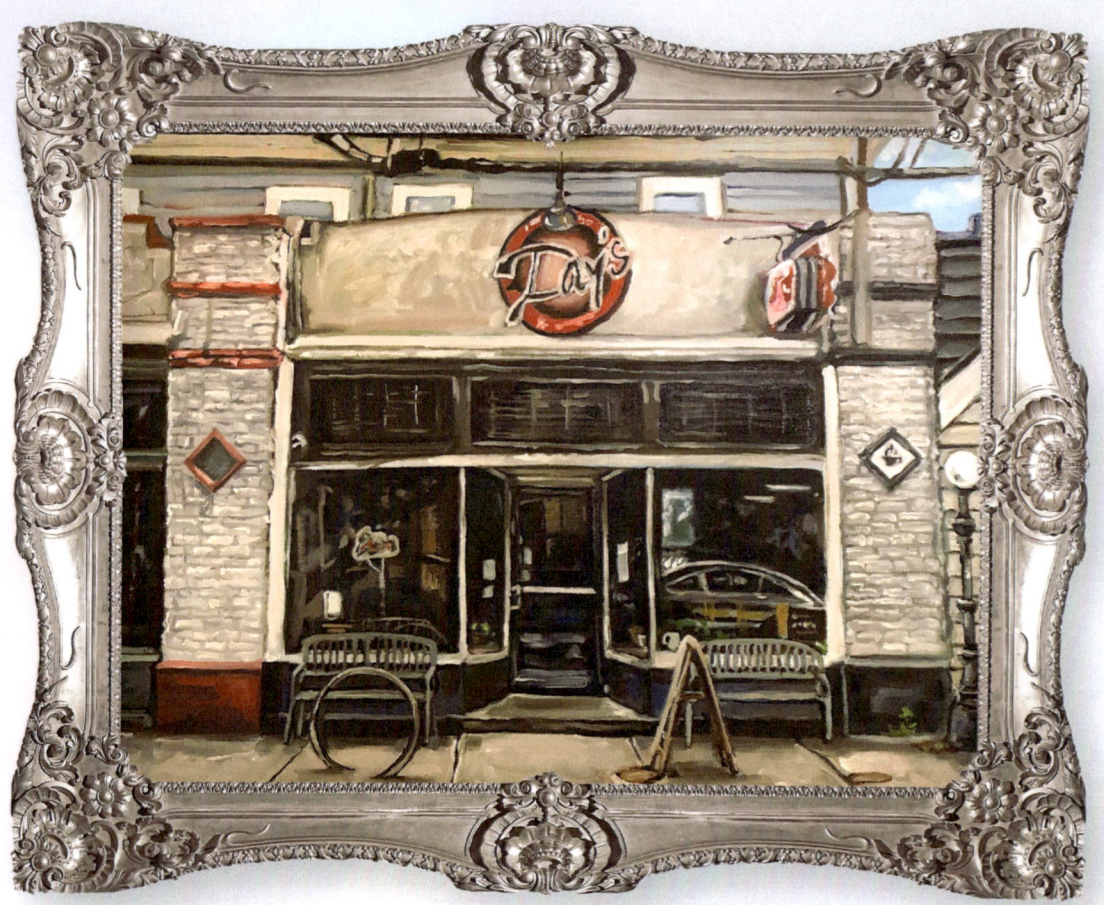

The crimson walls are lined with locally made art. There are people of all ages enjoying cappuccinos, hot chocolate, and each other at this beloved spot on Bardstown Road in the eclectic Highlands neighborhood.

Chris Roy started at Day's in 1995, a year after it opened. It was never highlighted as being specifically for LGBTQ+ folks, but it became a sacred meeting place for the community. "People even called us Gay's Coffee for a while," says Roy.

Roy is now a partner at Day's, where three of the four owners identify as LGBTQ+. A goal of his and the other owners is an inclusive, safe space, which is fostered partially by hiring people who they feel can provide that.

Roy reflects on Day's Coffee being 30 years old this year, alongside the Fairness Campaign turning 25, "Sometimes, I think we get caught up in the day to day, so it's easy to forget about the big picture. We are so, so proud. All we ever wanted to do was to feel like a space place, a home away from home."

Executive Director of the Fairness Campaign, Chris Hartman knows a thing or two about holding space for Queer folks in Kentucky. Hartman has helped pass anti-discrimination LGBTQ+ Fairness Ordinances in 21 Kentucky communities: from the state capitol to the small Appalachian town of Vicco.

"Day's has long been a safe haven and gathering spot for Queer folks in our community," says Chris Hartman. "As far back as I can remember, there were only a few places in town that I knew were reliably Queer—the clubs and Day's."

With safe spaces being few and far between for Queer folks, places to exist together were and are rare. This makes it difficult for community members to find and be with one another. Hartman recalls many first dates at Day's, as well as meetings for theater projects and the Fairness Campaign.

Carla Wallace, a co-founder of the Fairness Campaign, says that they knew from the beginning that they wanted to grow a movement. They shunned the 'behind closed doors' approach that she finds does not work in organizing. For Wallace, this was a chance to organize Queer people, but namely white Queer people, into a fight for liberation that centered racial justice.

The Fairness Campaign became a model of this approach to folks across the country, engaging thousands of people into the Queer, race, economic, and gender justice struggles. But, in order to engage a breadth of folks on a breadth of interconnected issues, Wallace says she knew that they needed to grow the movement.

"Being together in person is critical to movement building," she says. "Isolation puts us in danger, not only from potential violence, but from depression, addiction, and hopelessness."

For Wallace, spending time together in person is necessary to build community. But, in the same vein as what Hartman shares, Queer people have not historically had a lot of safe places to gather together.

With multiple Evangelical Christian backed and/ or owned coffee shops all around Louisville and the rest of the state, Day's has existed as an alternative. Having that safe space has been critical to movement building for Carla Wallace.

"We have to build across lines that those in power do not want us to build across," she says. "We cannot do that if we are in places where we cannot bring our full selves."

While there was a Fairness Office to hold meetings in, Wallace says they needed places with not just coffee, but good coffee.

She knew that Day's had Queer friendly owners, and it was a place they wanted to support. But, most importantly, Wallace knew she and her community would be welcomed.

Wallace notes the "great booths" at Day's, and how they spent hours there plotting—for the Fairness Campaign and for other community organizing. In those booths, there was strategy developed, but there was also a great trust sewn between the organizers: the foundation for movement building.

Wallace says we must have a "vision of collective liberation that leaves no one behind and has no illusions about a system that wants to let in only some of us—not all of us."

That vision is difficult to implement without being able to build it with others, especially when safe spaces are difficult to find. Roy shares that Day's hopes to be around for the next 30 years to continue being a safe space, a home away from home, and a place to not just get coffee, but good coffee.

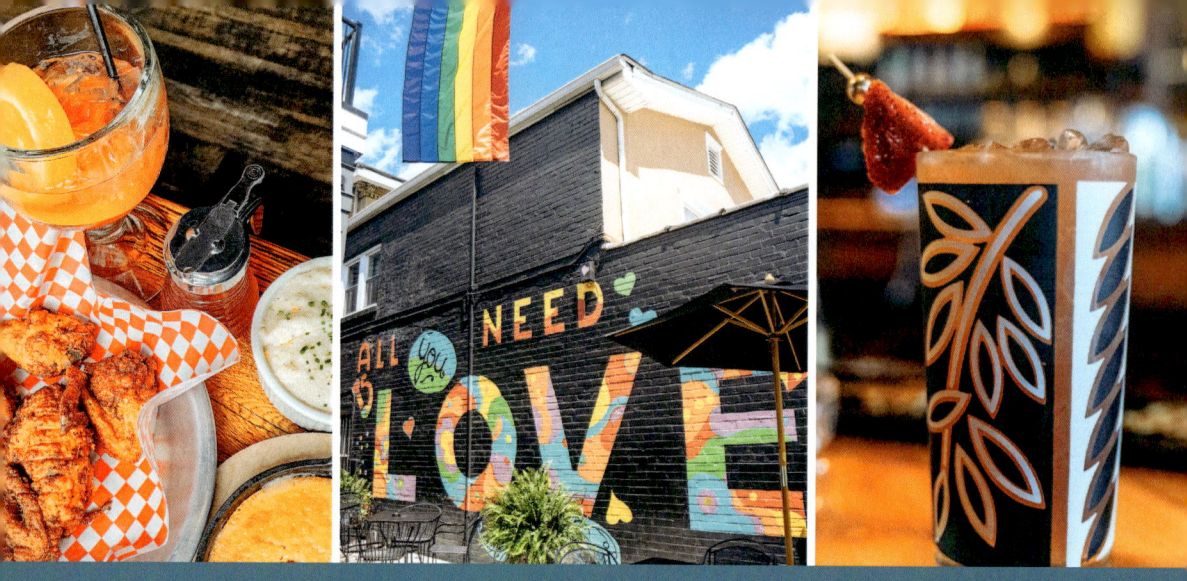

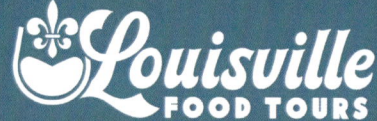

pride plates
QUEER HISTORY & FOOD TOUR

⏱ 3 Hours 🍴 5 Stops 📅 Wed – Fri 🕒 5-8 PM

louisvillefoodtours.com
use the code QUEERKY for 10% off

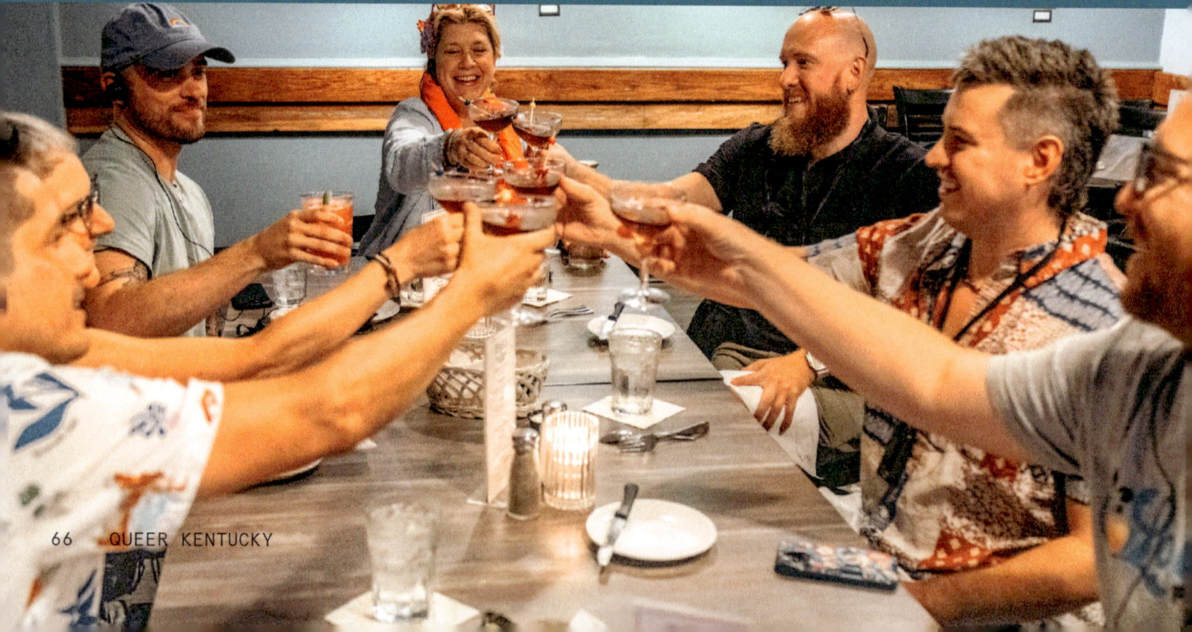

SUPPORT QUEER JOURNALISM

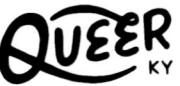

WWW.QUEERKENTUCKY.COM

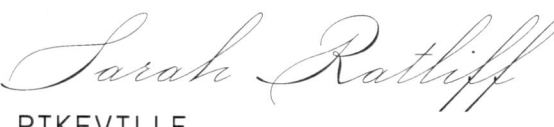

PIKEVILLE

she/her

Use one Queer slang word to describe Kentucky!

Kinky!

How did you activate and organize your community for equality?

I serve as board member Pikeville Pride and Main Street Pikeville and work constantly on creating community throughout Pikeville. This May, I presented at the Main Street Now national conference alongside other Pikeville Pride and Main Street members. Our presentation "Y'all Means All," details the story of Pikeville Pride and how we have gone from a small party in the city park to a full-fledged festival on Main Street. As Assistant Professor of Social Work at the University of Pikeville, I am faculty sponsor for Pride+, our campus LGBTQIA+ group.

In the last 25 years, what is one moment that gave you hope for Kentucky's fight in equality?

Seeing Andy Beshear at the Fairness Lobby Days at the Capital and then getting to shake his hand and thank him for his vocal support. Governor Beshear gives me hope that there ARE people in power in Kentucky who want equality.

What do you think is next for Kentucky in the fight for Equality?

I think we'll continue to see bigotry and hatred from those who are leading the anti-gay charge as they'll always find a new non-issue to focus on. My fear is the continuation of attacks on Queer families—adoption, fostering, marriage, family planning, medical coverage, etc.

What are Kentucky's greatest strengths when it comes to the fight for Queer equality?

Kentucky is filled with good people who truly want nothing but the best for their neighbors. While doing flood relief work in 2022, I saw so many people helping one another—some of them lost their own homes but worked tirelessly to muck out flooded houses owned by single moms, the sick, the elderly. That's true Kentucky selflessness—we can watch our home float down a river and immediately turn around and get back to work helping someone else.

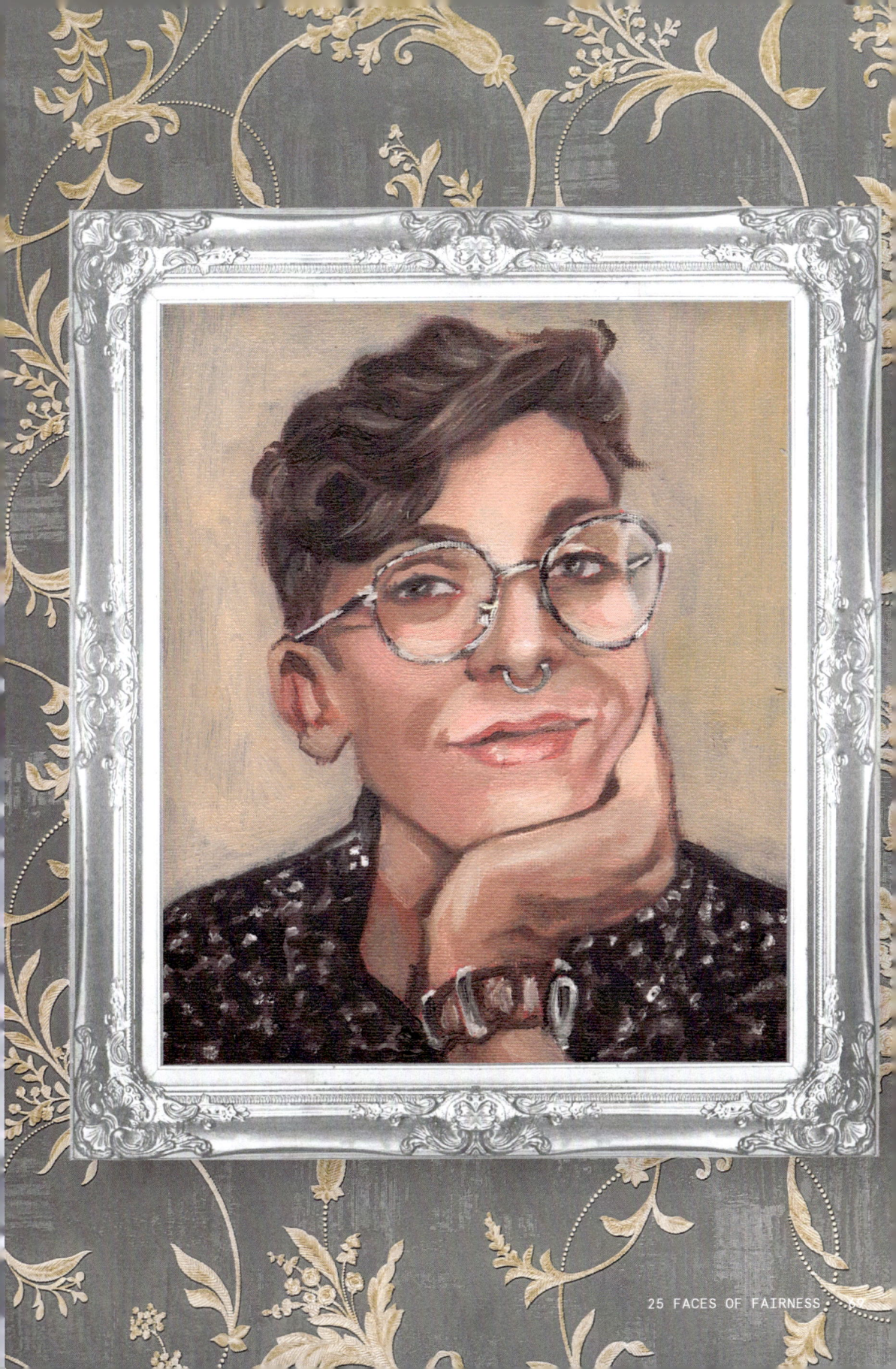

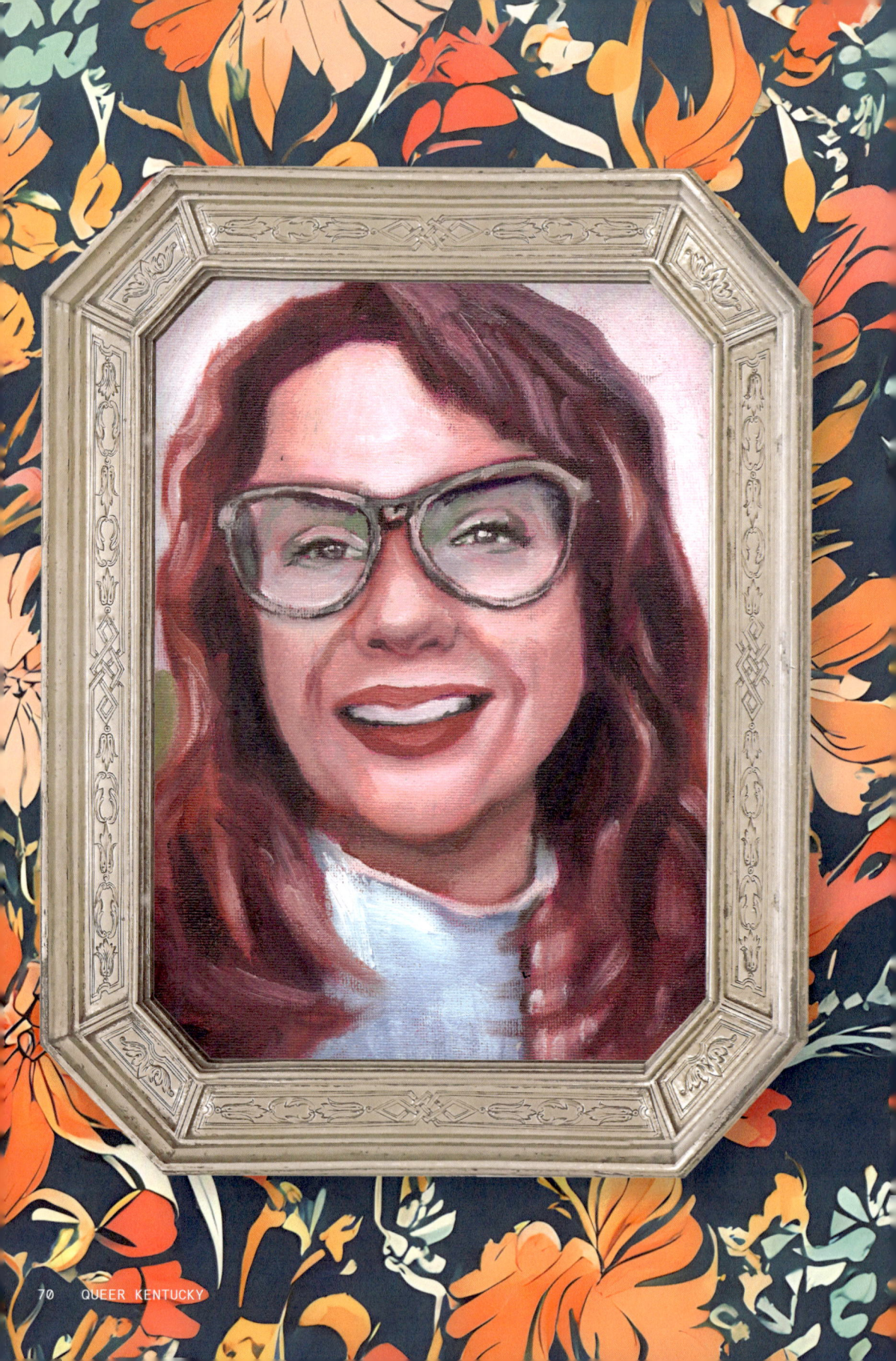

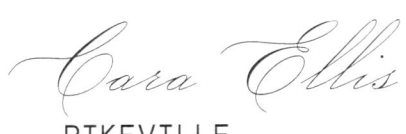

Cara Ellis
PIKEVILLE
she/her

Use one Queer slang word to describe Kentucky!

Folx - because as an Appalachian, I often address people as folks. It's in our blood! I also love the word camp/campy, as I feel like Kentucky is a wonderfully unique and kitschy place.

How did you activate and organize your community for equality?

I've been a community organizer for over five years, namely in the realm of LGBTQ+ and reproductive rights advocacy. Honestly, I got my start because I was passionate to see some change in my community. I didn't have a playbook per se to make change, I just threw myself out there and used social media as a platform to amplify my message. Social media can be a great tool in the fight for equality. Since 2018, I've been a member of Pikeville Pride, a local LGBTQ+ nonprofit dedicated to doing work in Eastern Kentucky. I currently serve as president, and our organization plans and hosts our annual Pride event in Pikeville. Last year, our event had over 2,300 attendees, which was our biggest to date. My work with Pikeville Pride has allowed me to talk to members of my community about the need to highlight the diversity and inclusion of LGBTQ+ in Appalachia because we're often overlooked or ignored. I like to tell folks we've here and we've always been here, and slowly but surely, we are putting a name to the faces of Queer folks in the region.

In the last 25 years, what is one moment that gave you hope for Kentucky's fight in equality?

Seeing a fairness ordinance being passed in Vicco gave me a lot of hope because if a small, rural town in Perry County can do it, to me, there is no reason we can't have a statewide fairness ordinance that not only helps protect Queer folks across the state, but other marginalized communities as well.

What do you think is next for Kentucky in the fight for Equality?

I see more cities, such as Pikeville, embracing a fairness ordinance and passing policy that protects our community. I also see LGBTQ+ organizations from across the state form a coalition to have a more visible presence in Frankfort to support programs and policies that will benefit our community.

What are Kentucky's greatest strengths when it comes to the fight for Queer equality?

Our greatest strength truly is our people. I've met some of the most dedicated advocates and organizers in my journey, including Carla Wallace, who has been involved in Queer advocacy in Kentucky for decades. The ones who paved the way for us to be where we are have welcomed the newer generation to continue the fight and given us the tools we need to succeed.

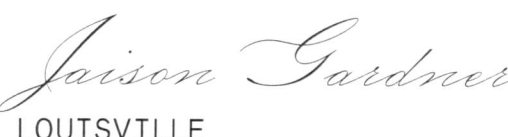

Jaison Gardner
LOUISVILLE
he/him

Use one Queer slang word to describe Kentucky!

Ovah!

How did you activate and organize your community for equality?

I have been active in the fight for equality since the mid 1990s. My activism has taken many forms but including as a leader or board member of local organizations including the Fairness Campaign and Sweet Evening Breeze (fun fact, I actually picked the name for the shelter/organization). I have also been a frontline activist, leading rallies and protests for equality. Lately I've used my work as a public speaker and podcaster to educate and inspire others to move on issues of justice. One of my proudest moments in recent years was co-organizing and leading a local memorial rally in response to the Orlando Pulse nightclub in 2016, that drew several thousand people to the big four Bridge.

In the last 25 years, what is one moment that gave you hope for Kentucky's fight in equality?

In 2013 the small Kentucky town of Vicco past a fairness ordinance. It is considered the smallest town in America with LGBTQ+ protections. This totally defied all the stereotypes that many people have about Kentucky, especially small town Kentucky. It was an inspiring moment to witness.

What do you think is next for Kentucky in the fight for Equality?

I think Kentucky will continue to be a quiet but consistent force in the fight for LGBTQ+ equality in the nation. I always like to tout the fact that Louisville had a trans inclusive comprehensive Fairness ordinance before many other cities and states in the nation, including New York City. The movement here locally has always held anti-racism as a primary tenet that informs that work we do and I think we can be a model for anti racist Queer liberation organizing.

What are Kentucky's greatest strengths when it comes to the fight for Queer equality?

So many experienced elders and so many inspiring new, younger activists. Folks doing organizing both in rural and urban parts of the state. A wonderful governor in Andy Beshear.

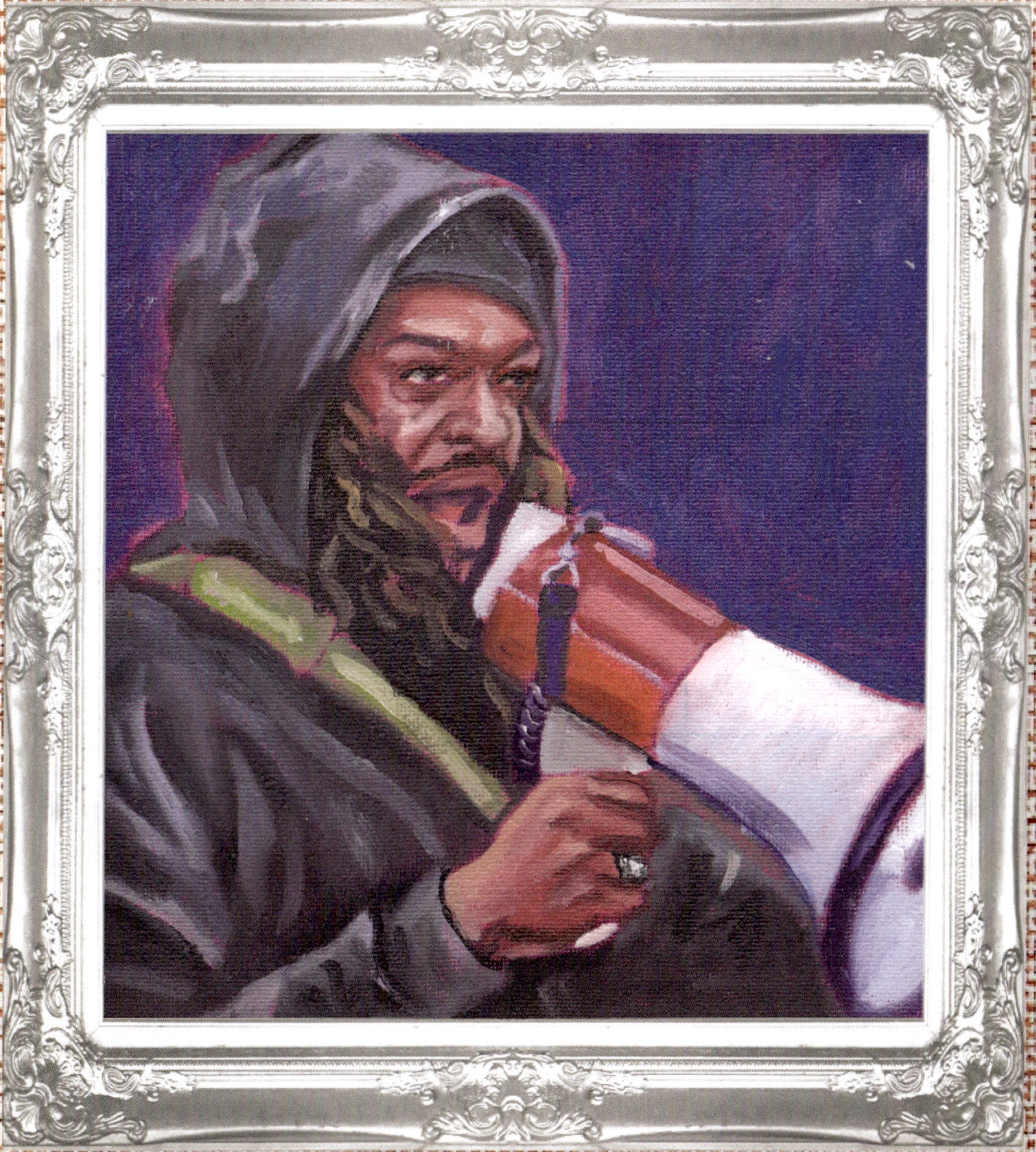

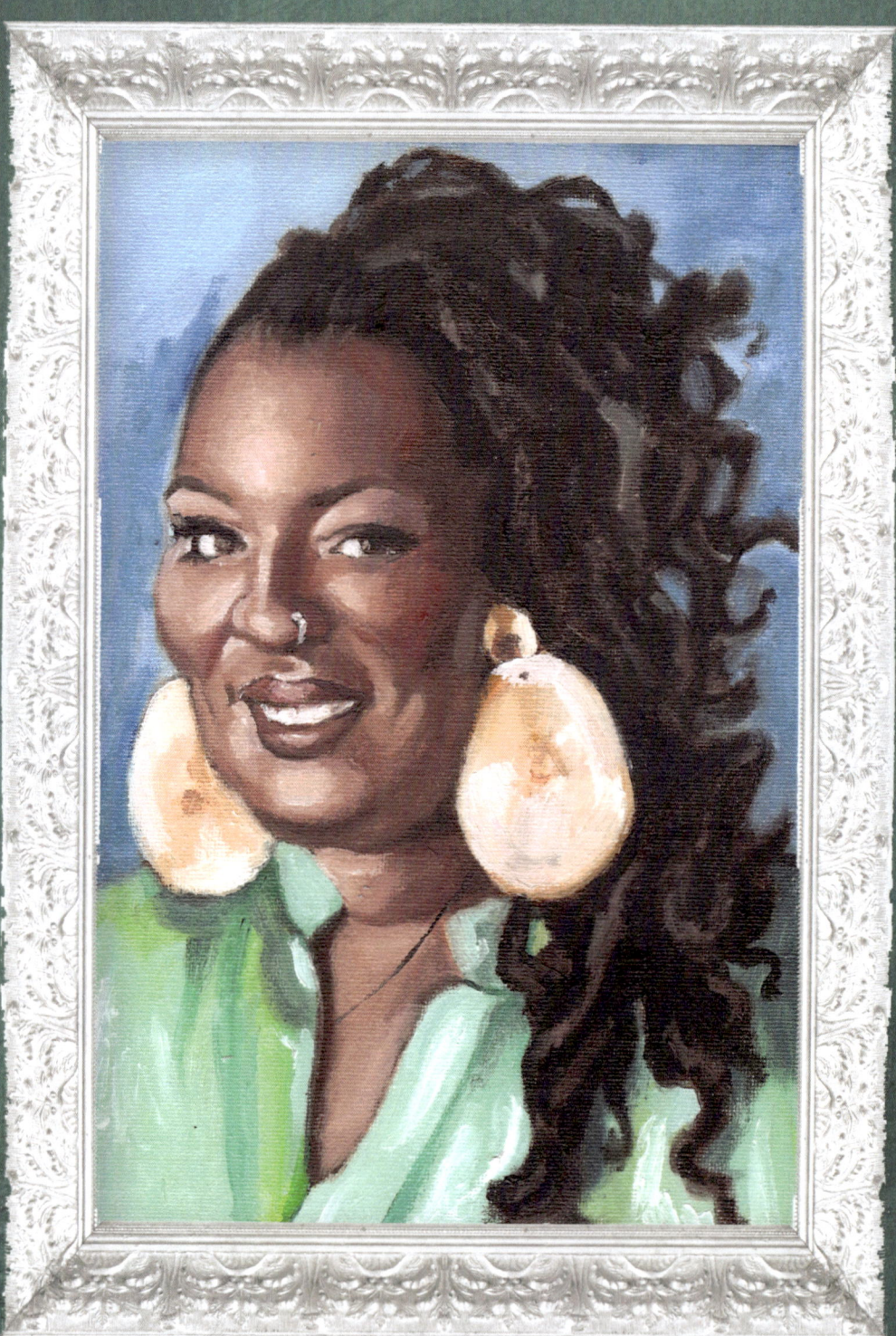

www.ingramcontent.com/pod-product-compliance
Lightning Source LLC
Chambersburg PA
CBRC101145030426
42337CB00009B/73